Sports Psychology in Action

Sports Psychology in Action

Richard J. Butler BSc, MSc, PhD, ABPsS, CPsychol
Consultant Clinical Psychologist, Leeds Community and Mental Health Trust, Consultant Sports Psychologist, British Olympic Association and Amateur Boxing Association, Honorary Lecturer, University of Leeds

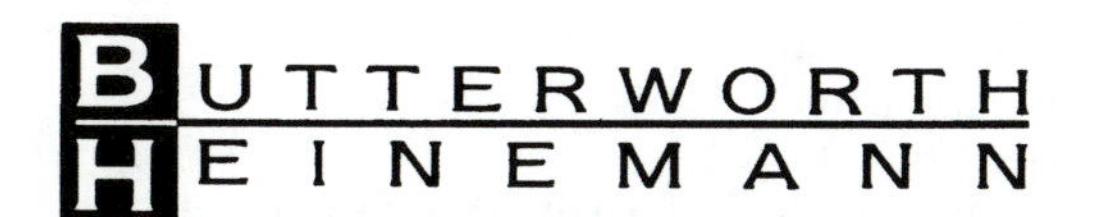

Butterworth-Heinemann Ltd
Linacre House, Jordan Hill, Oxford OX2 8DP

A member of the Reed Elsevier plc group

OXFORD LONDON BOSTON
MUNICH NEW DELHI SINGAPORE SYDNEY
TOKYO TORONTO WELLINGTON

First published 1996

British Library Cataloguing in Publication Data
A catalogue record for this book is available from the British Library

Library of Congress Cataloguing in Publication Data
A catalogue record for this book is available from the Library of Congress

ISBN 0 7506 2436 1

Typesetting and artwork origination by
David Gregson Associates, Beccles, Suffolk
Printed in Great Britain by Biddles Ltd, Guildford and King's Lynn

Contents

Acknowledgements

This book owes much to the efforts, enthusiasm and assistance of the following colleagues. I am grateful to Kevin Hickey who first encouraged and inspired me to apply some of my psychological thinking and approaches within sport. Ian Irwin has been particularly supportive and helpful in providing opportunities to develop these ideas, and along with Marcus Smith, has created a collaborative context whereby issues concerning performance enhancement have been effectively addressed. I am also grateful to Sarah Rowell for helping me keep abreast of current thinking and the Sports Council through the Sports Science Support Programme for their support in enabling me to apply psychological approaches at an elite level. I am indebted to Susan Devlin, my publisher, for her encouragement, vision and commitment to see the project completed. The efforts of Emma Hiley, Mandy Pullan and Julie Kemp have been crucial to the production of this book and I am duly indebted. Finally the book owes much to the many athletes with whom I have worked and I am grateful for their endeavour, patience and wisdom.

Although the male pronoun has been used throughout the text this is purely for simplicity and no bias is intended.

Dedicated to Sue, Joe, Gregory and Luke

1 Kick off: towards a model of psychology in sport

'The most powerful drive in the ascent of man is the pleasure of his own skill. He loves to do what he does well and, having done it well, he loves to do it better.'

J. Bronowski

If the ascent of man is a matter of intrinsic pleasure coupled with a need to achieve, the quest to perform well in a sporting context is, to paraphrase the late Bill Shankly, much more than this. Terry Orlick (1990) graphically describes what is at issue for the performer in the search for excellence, and the personal meanings which are confronted when the sporting arena is entered. They include:

- A sense of mastery – the feelings of grace, power, accuracy, speed and control of particular movements and skill.
- A sense of achievement – with executing a skill, accomplishing a specific tactical ploy, or following through a pre-planned routine.
- A search for perfection – to excel, perform consistently, improve, attain high standards, surpass previous personal bests.
- Delivering a statement about yourself – through style, creativity and expression.
- Putting yourself to the test – meeting a challenge, putting yourself on the line, testing your nerve, to grapple, struggle, to overcome the odds, to explore your potential, to be at the frontiers of the unknown.
- Drawing on reserves – to dig in, stretch yourself to the limit, to give all you have, to emerge invigorated.
- Sharing with others – the exhilaration of success, the acknowledgement of joint effort, the team culture, a drink in the bar afterwards.

Aspiring to excellence demands endeavour. An undertaking to address whatever it takes to achieve performances that test the athlete's potential. Metaphorically not to leave any stone unturned. A measure of performance effectiveness may be determined with reference to Peter Terry's (1989) formula which states:

Performance =	Physical preparation	+	Technical skill	+	Psychological readiness

This *triadic model* highlights the importance of preparation in all areas and predicts an inferior performance if any one aspect is neglected. Thus a gifted (technically skilled) player will underperform when either the physical or psychological preparation has not been fully addressed.

The extent and importance of the three factors seems dependent on:

- The national culture – e.g. the artistry, flamboyance and honed technique of football players from southern European countries compared with the fitness and work rate of those from northern European countries.
- The sport – some sports such as golf, fencing, archery and snooker tend to be technique-dominated whereas other sports like swimming, weightlifting, judo and squash balance technique with physical fitness.
- The individual – within the same sport some athletes will emphasize the importance of one attribute more than another but still seek to achieve the same level of performance. Thus batsmen in a cricket team may have widely contrasting styles, some depend on timing and technique while others rely on determination and concentration, yet all seek to mass the greatest number of runs they can.

Physical attributes are sometimes referred to as the **'Ss'**. They include:

Strength – e.g. weightlifting
Speed – e.g. sprinting
Stamina – e.g. long distance swimming
Suppleness – e.g. gymnastics

Technical attributes are sports specific but tend to rely on a foundation of:

Balance – e.g. ice skating
Eye hand co-ordination – e.g. shooting
Spring – e.g. high jump
Fluid movement – e.g. running
Orientation – e.g. diving
Reaction time – e.g. sprinting

Psychological attributes have been described as the **'Cs'**. They include:

Confidence
Concentration
Consistency
Control

Perhaps the most neglected area is that of psychological preparation. Below par performances are often characterized by failings of a psychological nature. Athletes 'choke under pressure', 'lack motivation', 'freeze at the starting line', 'become distracted', 'play without confidence', 'get the jitters' and so forth.

Terry Orlick and John Partington (1988) compared a group of athletes who performed well and exceeded their personal bests or expectations at the 1984 Olympic Games, with a group of athletes who did not perform to their usual standard. (The term 'athletes' is used throughout the book, in a generic sense, covering sports men and women from across a number of sports.) They concluded that the only factor distinguishing between the two groups was that the successful athletes had prepared psychologically.

What seems increasing veracious is the thoroughness of seeking mastery in physical and technical preparation, to a point where, at an elite level, there is not much to choose between athletes. What then emerges as significant is the degree to which the athlete has prepared psychologically.

Intriguingly, many athletes now acknowledge this:

'Marathon running, the toughest of all sports, is all in the mind.'
Chris Brasher

'Tennis is 80% head and 20% legs.'

Ion Tiriac (tennis coach)

'The most difficult area I work in is the position above the eyeballs.'

Tony Gray (rugby union coach)

'95% of the time it was psychological.'

Duncan Goodhew (swimmer)

'There were individuals in that race who were stronger, faster and more experienced, added to which, I was the slowest on paper, going into that final. There had to be factors other than physical ability which produced the end result.'

David Hemery (400m hurdle Olympic champion)

'Mental fitness is just about the most envied thing because it is the hardest to achieve and consequently the most difficult to break down when opposed by it.'

Angela Burton (tennis writer)

'90% of baseball is half mental.'

Jim Wohlford

'Putting is 70% technique, 30% mental.'

Mark James (golfer)

'Tennis is like a chess game and also an enormous physical contact of minds.'

John Newcombe

'You play from the shoulders up. It isn't all important, just 90%, and maybe over 90%.'

Arnold Palmer

'Once you've got the physical bit, then it's all in the mind.'

Nick Faldo

'For success, first, performers must have talent, second they must work and third they must have control of the mind.'

Valeriy Borzov (100m Olympic champion)

The psychological characteristics of successful performers has come under scrutiny. Work by Highlen and Bennett (1979) and

Mahoney and Avener (1977) has identified the following psychological skills. These might be construed as 'intuitive' skills as the athletes in question had discovered, without prior training and advice, the usefulness of the skills in enhancing their own performances. They are:

- the ability to control anxiety,
- being confident,
- the capacity to concentrate on the present,
- the use of imagery.

Since even top athletes have inconsistent performances, the notion of studying successful performers has given way to the analysis of successful performance. Inviting athletes to describe what characterizes their best or exceptional performances has led researchers like Ken Ravizza (1977), Garfield and Bennett (1984) and Gould, Eklund and Jackson (1922a, b) to identify the following:

- physically relaxed, in control, effortless performance;
- mentally relaxed, no fear of failure;
- confident, positive expectations;
- focused on the present, totally immersed in the activity, not distracted, detached from the external environment;
- highly energized;
- pre-competition preparation with visualization, mental rehearsal and planning.

With identification the question arises of how athletes might accomplish such skills to assist them in improving the quality and consistency of their performances. The idea of mental skills training was born; exercises for the athlete to practise, incorporate into training schedules and integrate, where possible, into their pre-match practice and performance.

John Syer (1989) has cultivated the concept that *all* physical, technical or mental exercises may, with some ingenuity, be employed to develop any physical, technical or mental skill. He uses a 3 × 3 matrix to elucidate this idea which he illustrates with an example from tennis (Figure 1.1), but which could equally be applied across all sports.

Tennis	Physical skills	Technical skills	Psychological skills
Physical training (weights)	Improves *strength*	Weights on wrist during practice improves the *volley*	Gradual increase in weights increases *confidence*
Technical training (feeding balls)	Non-stop to alternative sides improves *stamina*	To forehand improves the *stroke*	10 minute non-stop to forehand improves *concentration*
Psychological training (visualization)	A perfect half-volley improves timing	A perfect service improves *execution of the service*	A perfect service at game point improves ability to *deal with stress*

Figure 1.1 Syer's 3 × 3 model illustrating the interactional effects of training on the enhancement of physical, technical and psychological skills, with tennis. (Reprinted with the kind permission of Simon & Schuster)

If mental skills training is perceived as the focus of psychological intervention, this should not obscure the potential input of psychological involvement in a wider context. Variables such as character and strategy may have a critical influence in determining how an athlete performs, and these are no less psychological constructs than concentration or confidence. Figure 1.2 diagrammatically illustrates the variables recognized as important in the development of top performances. It depicts the physical, technical and psychological attributes linked and overlapping with co-ordination, strategy and character. It is those elements of a psychological nature – character and strategy – along with psychological skills which form the basis of this book. Chapters 4 to 14 deal with each aspect in turn. Chapter 2 provides essential reading in that it describes a method – performance profiling – of evaluating the perceived need of both coach and athlete. An underlying theme is one of understanding, which forms the basis for developing the subsequent techniques outlined in this book.

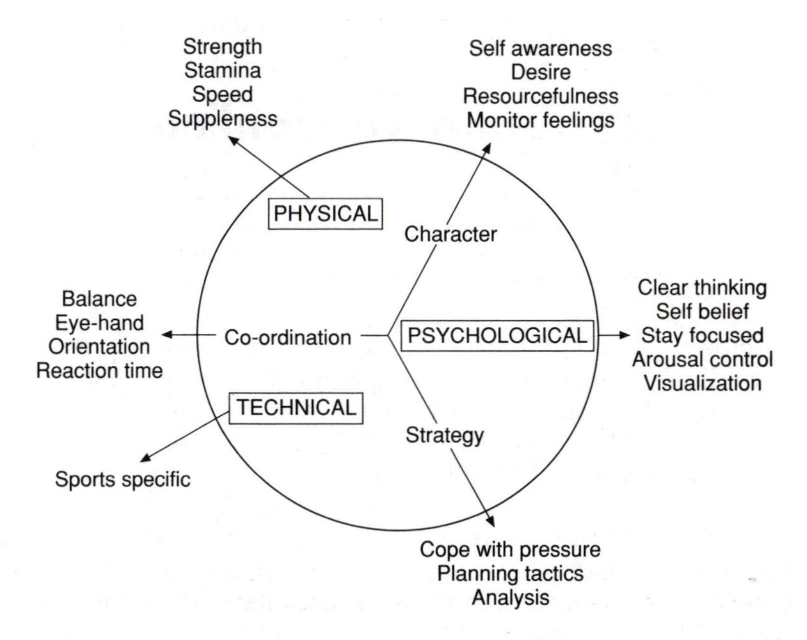

Figure 1.2 Model of attributes necessary for successful performance

A fundamental philosophy of the book is invitational. The techniques and exercises presented are for sampling, experimenting with, revising and adapting to your needs in probing for ways of enhancing the athlete's performance. In the final analysis reading and digesting will not be enough. Experimentation is a must. As Cus D'Amato, the illustrious boxing coach and mentor warned, 'It's not what a man says, but what he does at the end. That's what he intended to do all along.'

2 Performance profiling

'Perfection is not attainable, but if we chase perfection, we can catch excellence.'

Vince Lombardi

It remains an axiom that the athlete and coach view performance differently. An athlete will generally observe events from 'within'. The stride pattern, breathlessness, loss of rhythm, body temperature, the slippery surface underfoot, the signs of cramp, the pace of the ball, a pain in the shoulder and so forth. Typically a poor performance is attributed to incidents beyond their control and usually external to the athlete. Thus bad refereeing decisions, being beaten by a better person on the day, the difficult conditions or bad luck all take the blame for a poor showing.

In contrast, a coach characteristically observes from 'outside'. A trailing left leg, being out of position, lifting the head on contact, shuffling across the stumps and so forth. In addition, a below par performance is generally attributed by a coach to circumstances within the athlete's control such as a lack of effort, loss of form or not sticking to a pre-determined plan. Thus whereas an athlete tends to observe from within and attribute failure to events outside himself, the coach typically observes from outside and attributes poor performances to events within the athlete.

This paradox also surfaces in training. The athlete and coach may view training needs very differently. Traditionally it is the coach who takes the lead in planning and organizing a programme to strengthen weaknesses and ensure the athlete is in the best shape for the next competition. However the athlete may construe his needs in quite a different fashion, and where these are not accommodated, the result can lead to frustration, and 'switching off' thus nullifying any beneficial effects.

Performance profiling evolved as a method of increasing the coach's awareness whilst acknowledging the importance of the athlete's perspective. It is embedded in a psychological model, personal construct theory, which emphasizes each individual's unique way of making sense of the 'world'. Performance profiling illustrates the athlete's perceived strengths and weaknesses, described in terms meaningful to the athlete. This enhances the coach's understanding of the athlete, information the sensitive coach will take account of when designing a training programme.

Performance profiling thus leads to a more active participation on the athlete's behalf in decision making. It was developed as a means of helping coaches understand the athlete's needs and perspective (Butler, 1989), and is reviewed theoretically in the paper by Richard Butler and Lew Hardy (1992). It is now widely employed by sports scientists and coaches, usually as a first step in designing a training programme, whether the nature of that programme is aimed at developing physical, technical or psychological skills. Along with colleagues Marcus Smith and Ian Irwin, the author has described the way the performance profile can be used in practice (Butler, Smith and Irwin, 1993).

Three intentions are raised by employing the performance profile:

- It is an invitation to consider the athlete's view or perspective, thus encouraging the sharing of information and needs.
- It establishes notions of what the athlete considers important in order to perform well, thus raising awareness.
- It encourages training and coaching tailored to meet the needs of the athlete.

The benefits of using the performance profile are as follows:

- a visual display of the athlete's evaluation,
- it engages the athlete in an assessment of qualities needed to perform consistently well,
- the athlete's views can be matched with that of the coach,
- it establishes the important areas to work on,
- it enables progress to be monitored,

- it provides a way of analysing performance following competition.

Graham Jones (1993) has commented that the performance profile commits the athlete to the training programme given their investment in evaluating their needs, and the technique is also a way of testing the effectiveness of any intervention or programme designed to help the athlete.

The steps required to develop a performance profile are as follows:

- identify the qualities or attributes the athlete thinks are necessary in order to achieve a top performance,
- encourage the athlete to rate themself (how they are at present) on each quality.

Identify the important qualities

> 'A cricketer needs stamina, speed, strength, agility, a keen eye, a strong individual initiative, team spirit, cool judgement and fast reflexes.'
>
> *Sir Gary Sobers*

Table 2.1 A sample of the types of qualities to emerge when analysing the performances of top athletes

Physical	*Co-ordination*
Strong, stamina, endurance, suppleness, fit, quick, sharp, agile, powerful, explosive	Balance, reactions, eye-hand co-ordination, rhythm, flow, recovery rate
Technical	*Strategy*
Sports specific	Planning, tactics, setting targets, goals, cope with pressure
Psychological	*Character*
Confident, focused, control nerves, ability to relax, regain focus, visualization	Weight control, competitive, dedicated, will to win, disciplined, enjoy training, determined

The customary way of identifying qualities is to ask the athlete their opinion of what attributes make up a top performance. This, of course, can be undertaken as a group or team exercise with members 'brainstorming' the important qualities. Each member of the team would then need to select what is important for them from the numerous qualities generated. Sometimes, as a prompt, the athlete might be encouraged to think of another athlete who excels at the sport, or produces performances he wishes to emulate, and then envisage what qualities or assets they possess.

A further prompt should stimulate the athlete to gather a selection of qualities from each of the physical, technical, psychological, co-ordination, strategy and character domains. Table 2.1 provides examples of possible qualities.

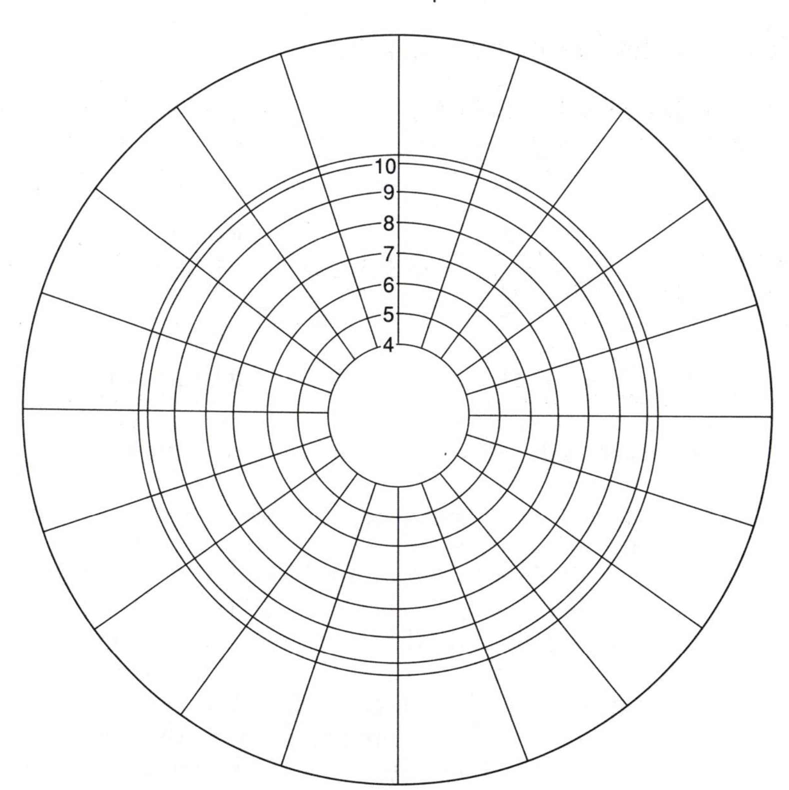

Figure 2.1 Blank performance profile

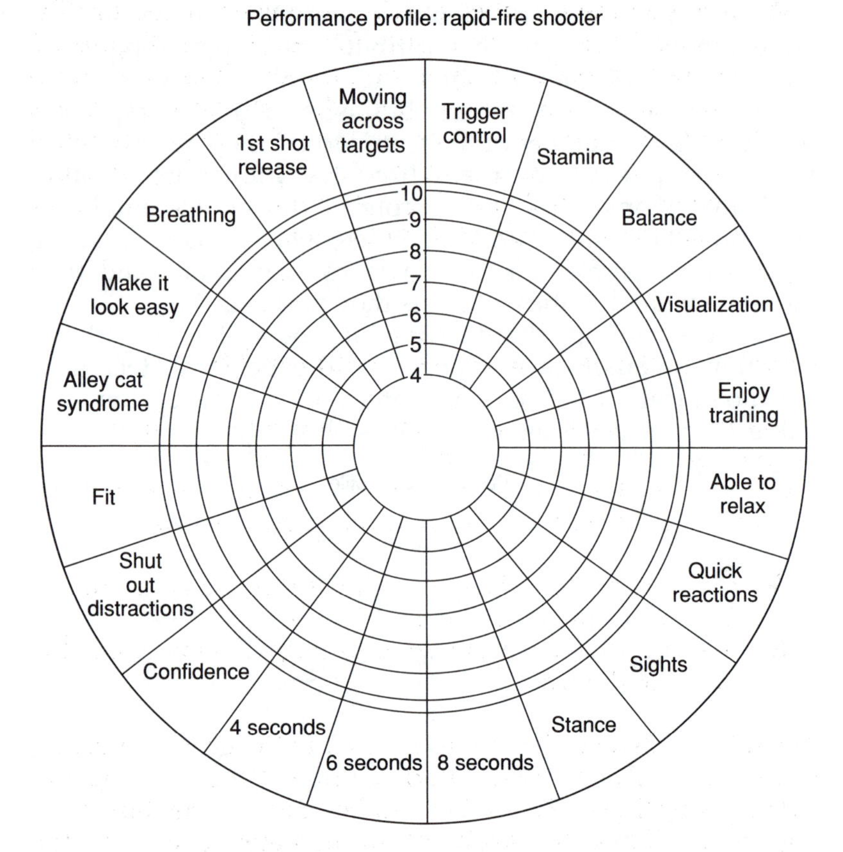

Figure 2.2 Qualities of a rapid-fire shooter displayed on the profile

When undertaking this venture it is important to:

- Recognize there are *no* right or wrong answers – each response is a valid statement made by the athlete.
- There is no limit to the number of qualities elicited by the athlete, but subsequently a selection of the twenty most important should be made in order to fit on the profile. More than one profile may of course be used to accommodate a wide range of qualities.
- Use the labels or descriptions given by the athlete. To avoid misunderstanding ask the athlete to define what is meant by each quality.

- Arrange the qualities on the perimeter of the profile. Figure 2.1 is a blank profile for you to use. Figure 2.2 shows a profile incorporating the qualities of a rapid-fire shooter. Note this includes physical attributes (stamina, fitness), co-ordination (balance), technical skills (sights, first shot release), psychological competence (confidence, visualization), and character (enjoy training, alley cat syndrome).

Invite athlete to rate self on each quality

This helps to formulate a picture of perceived strengths and weaknesses. Using a rating scale from 0 (not at all) to 10 (very much so), ask the athlete to judge his present level on each quality as he perceives it *now*. The only adjoiners are:

- that not too long is spent deliberating or analysing as this makes the rating more difficult,
- that the athlete should be encouraged to maximize the range of the scale.

The ratings then need to be transferred to the profile. A rating of 10 is represented by the outermost ring, 9, the next ring and so on. Scores lower than 4 have to be noted in the 'bullseye'. Figure 2.3 shows the profile of an amateur boxer with the ratings shaded in to provide a visual map of his perceived strengths and weaknesses. This profile also includes the boxer's rating of where he would ideally wish to be, which is illustrated with a dotted line. The profile in Figure 2.3 indicates that the boxer rates himself highly on character (competitive, determined) and on most physical attributes other than suppleness, reasonably high on strategy (switch tactics) and co-ordination (reactions) and relatively low on most technical attributes and the one psychological quality, that of confidence. This then provides a clear indication of the boxer's needs which will prove invaluable to the coach in designing an appropriate training programme.

The performance profile is a flexible instrument. Some additional uses it can be put to include: (i) assessing the

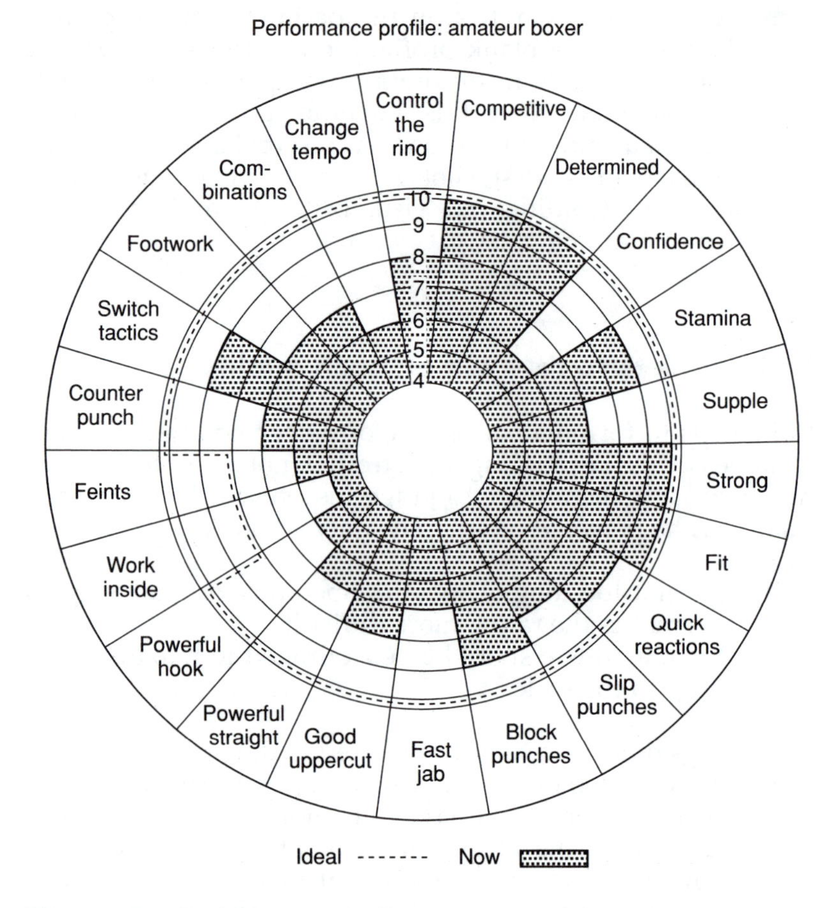

Figure 2.3 Performance profile of an amateur boxer

discrepancy between athlete and coach, (ii) arriving at a benchmark, (iii) monitoring progress.

Assessing the discrepancy between athlete and coach

This entails the coach rating his view of the athlete on the same qualities, preferably without previous knowledge of how the athlete has rated himself. When the two ratings

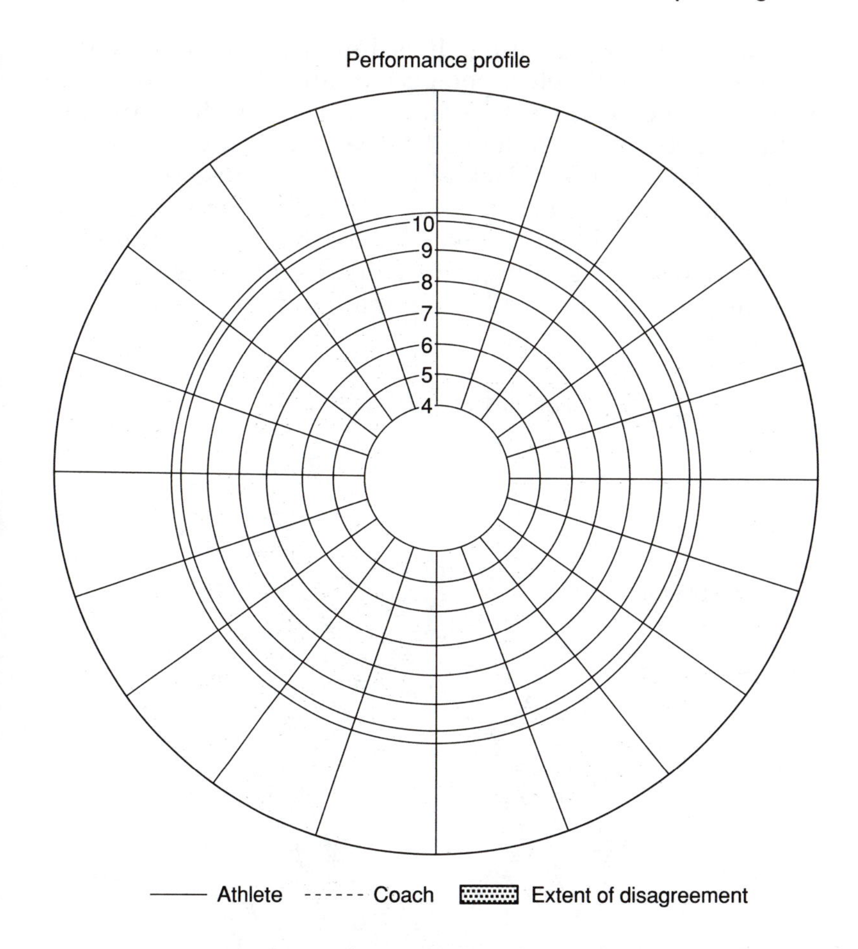

Figure 2.4 Blank profile for use in assessing the degree of mismatch between athlete and coach

(athlete and coach) are plotted on the profile, the similarity of ratings can readily be seen. Figure 2.4 is a blank profile designed to accommodate both ratings, with the difference between ratings being shaded in. A close correspondence between athlete and coach suggests the basis of a good working arrangement as they are both 'on the same wave-length' with respect to the athlete's needs. Large discrepancies between athlete and coach should lead to a discussion about the reasons for each rating. It is important that the coach understands the athlete's perspective and does not override or devalue the athlete's assessment. It is often these areas of 'mismatch' between athlete and coach which accounts for fraught relationships or lack of progress, because they are at odds in how they construe what is needed. Sometimes it is helpful for the athlete to take the coach's stance in understanding the coach's rating, and video feedback, when available, can prove dramatically illuminating in this respect.

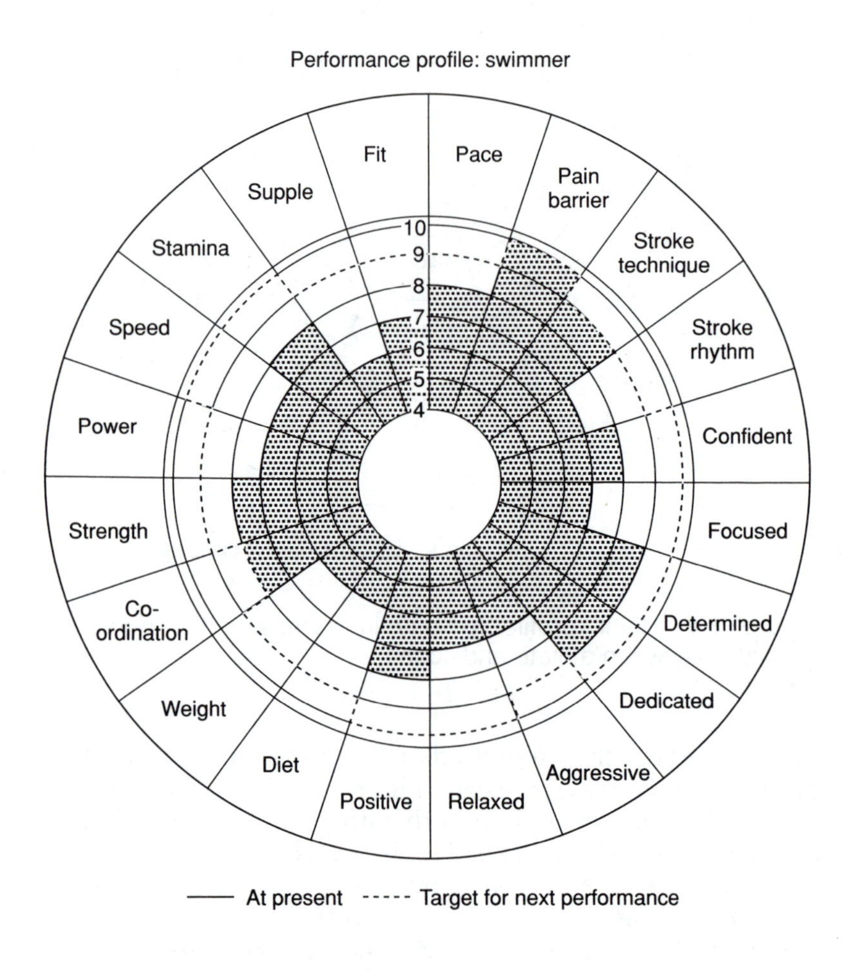

Figure 2.5 Performance profile of a swimmer

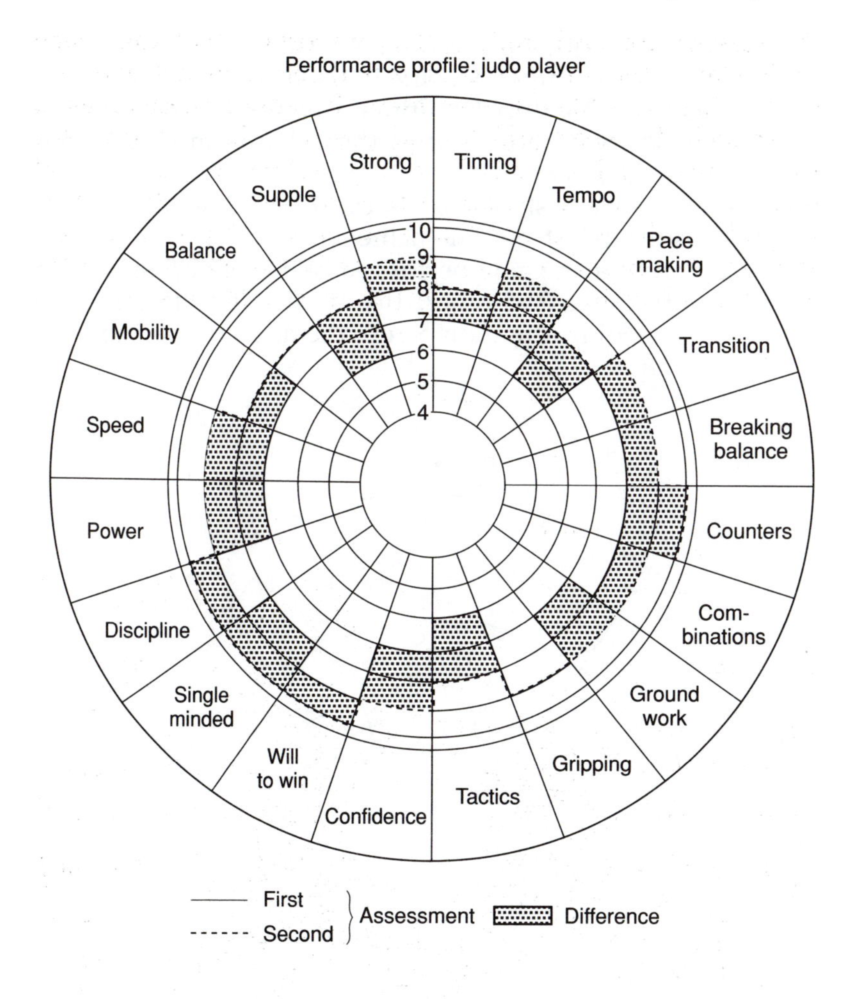

Figure 2.6 Performance profile of a judo player

Arriving at a benchmark

Fundamentally this refers to where the athlete would wish to be. It may involve:

- An ideal (how I would like to be). As Figure 2.3 shows this rating would normally and expectedly be a '10' which describes perfection. Any ratings less than 10 immediately suggest some resistance on the athlete's behalf to achieving the ultimate. For example, it may be that quality is construed by the coach as important but not by the athlete.

- A previous best performance. This provides a more realistic target to seek to achieve.
- A target for the next performance. Figure 2.5 shows an example of a swimmer, the profile highlighting the areas needing attention before the next competition.

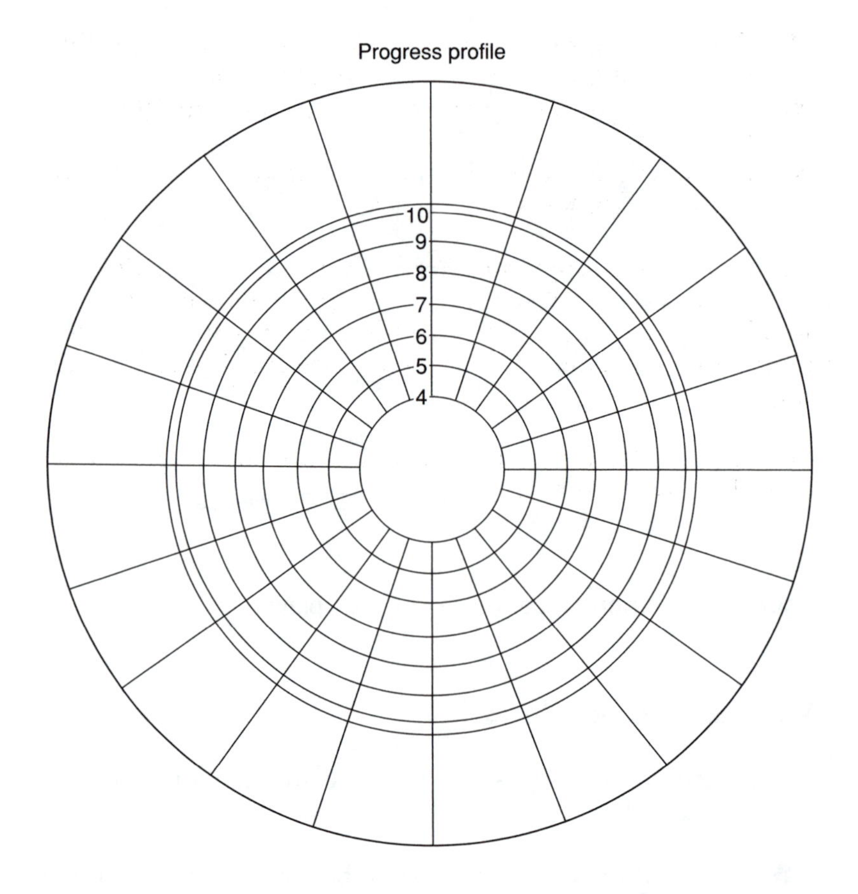

Figure 2.7 Blank profile for use in monitoring progress

Monitoring progress

Subsequent assessments over a period of time will provide a measure of progress. Figure 2.6 shows the progress made by a judo player over the course of a training camp. Such signs of progress instil confidence in athletes and serve to inform the coach of the effectiveness of the training programme. Figure 2.7 is a blank progress profile for use in monitoring. Signs of a lack of progress require investigating in a similar invitational style used to explore differences between coach and athlete ratings. The following possibilities may account for a lack of progress:

- the athlete has no investment in the quality, suggesting the attribute was imposed by someone else,
- the quality is perceived as not required for the next performance,
- the coaching programme did not address the issue, or failed to help the athlete improve.

Performance profiling is an adaptable technique, assisting the coach in an ever-increasing need to understand the athlete. It should set the scene for designing an appropriate training programme and help to monitor the athlete through to the competition.

> 'Mohammed Ali was so quick he would click off the light and be in bed before the room got dark.'
>
> *George Foreman*

3 Maximizing training

'The more I practise the luckier I become.'

Gary Player

The good coach, like the good athlete, is in constant pursuit of improvement, searching for more effective techniques to enhance the quality of training sessions. This may take the form of innovative techniques, better communication or changes in coaching style. Whatever the new idea, it requires a foundation of good practice. Without structure, training becomes piecemeal and ineffective. This chapter explores the psychological side of training sessions by considering those factors which can play an important part in ensuring sessions are effective.

A starting point is an assessment of the athlete's view of what characterizes an effective training session. Athletes claim to achieve more in a climate where the coach:

Informs
Involves
Inspires

The coach who **informs**:

- *Plans* and *publishes* sessions in advance. Athletes are then prepared, knowing what to expect, and while coaches may still at times have to 'think on their feet', a basic format can be followed which links to an overall programme designed to bring the athlete to his peak.
- Starts and ends sessions on *time*. This again meets the athlete's expectations and encourages concentration throughout the session.
- Lets the athletes know the *aim* of the session. This spells out what the session is designed to achieve and what the athlete will 'take away' with him.

- Provides *clear reasons* for the method selected to achieve the aim.
- Gives *clear instructions*.
- Provides a *range of input*.

Effective coaching utilizes instruction, modelling and questioning to help the athlete focus on the task.

Instructions should be precise and constructive. Avoid prefacing any instruction with *'don't'* (e.g. 'don't drop your shoulder') as this tends to remind the athlete to drop his shoulder. It focuses attention on what the athlete is not supposed to do, and by contrast does not inform the athlete of what is necessary and required in order to improve on the skill or technique.

Modelling might involve demonstration or video example, and it is essential to direct the athlete's attention towards the important elements of the performance.

Questioning should help the athlete raise awareness of how he currently performs a skill, what is perceived to be incorrect and what the perfect performance would feel like

> 'I've trained twelve years in order to experience these feelings of winning which last about twenty seconds.'
>
> *Adrian Moorhouse*

The coach who **involves**:

- Provides *variety* within and between sessions.
- *Individualizes* his methods to suit each athlete.
- Encourages *immediate* goals.

A method Ken Ravizza (1987) uses when athletes find it difficult to maintain concentration is the *two-minute focus*. This involves encouraging the athlete to focus completely on the task for just the next two minutes. This can break the tendency to be distracted and helps the athlete to become fully engaged again.

> 'The great joy days were the training days.'
>
> *Ron Pickering*

The coach who **inspires**:

- Provides *competition* or *challenges* to reach a target.
- Provides *feedback* during the session.
- *Evaluates* the sessions once it has finished.

> 'Everyone has a will to win but few have a will to prepare to win.'
>
> *Vince Lombardi*

The will to prepare is encouraged by training sessions which incorporate the following:

Goal setting
Emphasis on quality
Feedback
Evaluation
Rest

Setting a goal

> 'By having a definite plan to follow you feel that each ten-mile run through the rain is a specific piece of the jigsaw, not just another run.'
>
> *Brendon Foster*

Robert Weinberg (1994) suggests a goal is simply defined as what the individual is consciously trying to do. It seems undeniable that most athletes will make their own goals where none are made explicit. Such 'internal' goals however pose a problem. They may not necessarily be appropriate for developing a particular skill, and being unknown to the coach, they may cut across the aims of a training session. Goals then are best developed by both coach and athlete. They are also best tailored to each individual's needs. When developing goals the following points seem pertinent:

- Identify an area to work on. The performance profile will immediately highlight where this might be. Qualities to be considered are those where there is:
  - a perceived weakness where the athlete gives himself a low rating;

  - a discrepancy between the self and ideal rating, which as Garland (1985) suggests is the image of a future level of performance the individual wishes to achieve;
  - a discrepancy between the coach and athlete's rating on a particular quality.
- Identify what can be done to facilitate improvement on the quality. This should always aim to describe what is expected as it is the anticipation of achieving this which moves or excites the athlete to tackle the task. The description should seek to be as illustrated in Table 3.1:

Table 3.1 Examples of strong and weak descriptions of goal behaviour

Setting goals	
Phrased positively	*Not negatively*
✓Develop a top spin lob	✗Don't overhit the lob
✓Change tempo	✗Stop being one paced
✓Improve returns to wicket keeper	✗Reduce wild throws
Performance tasks	*Not outcome*
✓Chip at the flag	✗Finish in the top three
✓Head downwards at goal	✗Win each frame
✓Hit the board	✗Keep par for each hole
Controllable	*Not outside your control*
✓Plan a final effort	✗Force my opponent into errors
✓Develop height on the service throw	✗Get the crowd behind me
✓Visualize the jump before attempting	✗Trap more batters lbw
Specific	*Not global*
✓Breathe out on the backswing	✗Improve my discipline record
✓Hit the bottom corner with a penalty	✗Be a better defensive player
✓See the ball go into the pocket before each shot	✗Become more aggressive
Achievable	*Not unrealistic*
✓Achieve 50% success with free throws	✗Aim for 100% penalty saves
✓Get 70% of first serves in	✗Go for the maximum score
✓Run the last 400 m in 62 seconds	✗Beat the record

Phrased positively – avoiding negative statements which describe what not to do.
Performance tasks – Burton (1989) suggests tasks are more effectively accomplished when described in terms of behaviours needed to accomplish them, than when described as outcomes.
Controllable – the task has to be something the athlete can work on.
Specific – Richard Cox (1995) points out that too often athletes attempt to make gross changes in their performance, and thereby fail to concentrate on the specifics of performance which are more accessible to change.
Achievable – Goal setting theory suggests difficult tasks lead to higher performance but this has not been shown to be necessarily true for sports people. It seems important that the task is meaningful, challenging and designed along with the athlete to commit his investment.

'When you set your aim too high and don't fulfil it, then your enthusiasm turns to bitterness. Try for a goal that's reasonable, and then gradually raise it. That's the only way to get to the top.'
Emil Zatopek

Having made a goal, check the description against the following points before working on it:

- Is it positive?
- Does it describe what has to be done?
- Do I have control over making it happen?
- Is it described in sufficient detail?
- Can I reasonably be expected to carry it out?

An affirmative answer to each question suggests a workable task. The advantages of having goals to work on include (i) they keep the athlete focused on what is required; (ii) they provide and clarify direction; (iii) they increase determination and persistence to achieve the task; and (iv) they increase confidence when tasks and goals are achieved.

Goals and the tasks designed to achieve the goal require monitoring. If the tasks are proving too difficult they may need specifying in more detail. When they are accomplished; it is time to set another. As Jack Nicklaus commented, 'In golf you are always breaking a barrier. When you bust it, you set yourself a little higher barrier and try to break that one'.

Quality

Quality is really making it count. It is the antithesis of stultifying repetitions and going through the motions. Training sessions with an accent on quality are marked by realism, perfection and effort expended on difficult-to-master skills.

Realism

> 'Practice without reference to playing the full game produces "circus performers".'
>
> *Len Hoy* and *Cyril Carter* (basketball)

This refers to making the sessions as close to the competitive situation as possible and it might include wearing the appropriate kit, warm-up routines and psychologically preparing for the session. Geoff Boycott noted that 'You only instil good habits by taking practice seriously', suggesting that what is learnt in practice is what is transferred to competition. Where possible it is helpful to simulate the specifics of a competition or venue by holding sessions to mimic the event. Thus audio tapes of hostile crowds might be played, or stooge referees employed to set up difficult scenarios for the athletes to familiarize themselves with. Some athletes try to visualize the competitive arena during training sessions as Al Oerter explains 'I can mentally picture myself competing with other people in a training session'.

Perfection

> 'If I'm going to take the energy to practise, it's got to count. I'm better off doing four perfect exercises than doing twenty that are just mediocre.'
>
> (Successful Olympic gymnast)

Accomplishing a task, routine or technique once is far better than getting it nearly right many times. Limiting the number of repetitions tends to focus the athlete's thinking, as Ken Ravizza (1987) suggests, on the experience – the awareness of muscular tension, balance and so forth – in contrast to massed practice which engineers the habit of going through the motions. Whereas quantity refers to perhaps practising the same stroke or shot a hundred times, quality refers to the attempt to perfect and experience the shot a few times.

Effort expended on difficult-to-master skills

Four methods are described which can assist the athlete to develop techniques which are proving difficult to accomplish. These are discussed in depth by John Syer and Chris Connolly (1984).

1 Practise with *eyes closed*:
- first practise a skill with eyes open,
- then practise the same skill a number of times with eyes closed,
- concentrate on how the action feels,
- notice which muscle groups stretch,
- try again with eyes open.

2 Practise in *slow motion*:
- slow the movement right down,
- notice what happens and correct any faults at that speed,
- become aware of what the movement feels like,
- gradually increase the speed of movement,
- quicken it to the desired pace without altering the technique.

> 'Learn to use slowness to your advantage.'
>
> *Michael Stich*

3 Notice *breathing patterns*:
- whilst practising a skill become aware of when you inhale, hold and exhale,
- notice the levels of muscular tension as you do this,
- try altering your breathing pattern so you breathe in when you normally exhale and breathe out when you normally inhale,
- notice how your breathing pattern alters the execution of the skill,
- notice what improves the skill. (Usually exhaling as you execute a skill will reduce tension.)

4 Practise in your mind's eye:
- following the successful execution of a movement or technique close your eyes and picture yourself accomplishing the task,
- focus on how your muscles moved and stretched,
- run through the successful movement a number of times; this will imprint the action in memory.

Feedback

> 'There is a world of difference between what a diver thinks he is doing and what he is doing.'
>
> *Wally Orner* (diving coach)

Feedback is the provision of information about a performance. It can take a variety of forms:

- *Knowledge of results.* The familiar comments made by observers is an example of this. Such feedback, for maximum effect, should be delivered immediately following the action or skill. If corrections are required to the skill, the instructions should follow some positive comments about the performance.
- *Objective measures.* Can the athlete's performance be measured in terms of time, distance, power, strength or accuracy. Immediate feedback serves to raise awareness while keeping a diary of performances can provide a valuable record of progress.
- *Self monitoring.* This might include monitoring the action, or the effects of the action. Inviting the athlete to take note of what he feels during the execution of a skill directs attention to kinaesthetic or muscular changes. In this way tension, for example, can be located. In addition the athlete can be asked to consider the effect of his action and so, for example, listen to the sound of a ball hitting the racket, an oar entering the water or feet pounding the ground. In this way distinctive sounds become linked to successful actions which inform the athlete if errors creep into the performance.

- *Snap judgements.* Tim Gallwey (1974) advocated the athlete rating his own actions. The task is initially set, which might consist of a technique – a left uppercut, a feint to the right, a fast yorker, a bunker shot – or a description of the desired performance – relaxed, smooth, fast, powerful. With perfect execution deserving a rating of 10, the athlete rates his performance after each attempt.
- *Video playback.* The steps involved in using video for feedback include: (i) an agreement to focus on one aspect of the performance (which might have been highlighted through previous video analysis); (ii) video a short sample of the performance; (ii) before watching the replay, encourage the athlete to analyse the performance and rate it out of 10; (iv) when watching the playback observe and comment on the accuracy of the athlete's analysis and rating.

The benefits of feedback include raising the athlete's awareness, focusing attention, offering a challenge and enhancing confidence when performances are surpassed.

Evaluation

Following a training session an evaluation conducted by both athlete and coach can prove helpful in preparing for future sessions. The salient questions to address are:

- What went well?
- What requires changing?

Rest

> 'There is a time to run and there is a time to rest. It is the true test of the runner to get them both right.'
>
> *Noel Carrol* (Olympian and writer)

Athletes rest to aid recovery between bursts of activity and between training sessions. Quick recovery between activities can be assisted by a technique known as centering. Centering increases oxygen uptake by lowering the diaphragm and expanding the lungs. It involves:

- standing with feet apart and knees bent slightly,
- relaxing the neck and shoulders,
- breathing in through the nose and pushing the stomach *out*, keeping the neck and shoulders relaxed,
- holding in for a few seconds,
- exhaling slowly through the mouth,
- repeating this process 4–6 times.

Recovery between sessions can be helped by relaxation (see also Chapter 11), massage, swimming, sauna or a spa. Sleep is a more obvious choice but many athletes find difficulty in getting off to sleep. A favoured way of inducing sleep is to:

- Concentrate on feeling *heavy*. So heavy that the muscles feel like dropping through the bed (this relaxes the muscles).
- Develop a *shallow* breathing pattern.
- *Imagine* a small coloured (blue) dot against a background of contrasting colour (green). Picture the small dot very slowly and gradually expanding in size until it consumes the total visual field. (Usually sleep occurs before the background is fully covered.)

Prolonged and intensive training can lead to what is termed 'over training', a condition which makes it increasingly difficult for the athlete to engage in and benefit from further training. The perceptive coach will remain vigilant for signs that the athlete is becoming stressed by training. Such signs include a worsening or increase in:

- sore muscles,
- stiffness,
- disturbed sleep,
- poor appetite,
- persistent tiredness,
- feeling weak
- slow reactions,

- feeling fed-up and moody,
- slow recovery between sessions,
- short tempered and irritable,
- lack of effort in training.

Typically, when overtraining is suspected, the advice is to reduce training loads and encourage recovery through relaxation, sauna, massage and sleep. Overtraining might also be seen as a symptom of a training programme too forceful in design. It is thus a time for reflection and restructuring of the programme to ensure training sessions are maximized. As Douglas Wakiihuri, the famous marathon runner said, 'Preparation must be all as one. You need to run, to recover, to eat, to have shoes.'

4 Self awareness

'Self awareness is the most important thing towards being a champion.'

Billie Jean King

A perennial issue for those working with athletes is to understand what makes them 'tick'. To fathom out what is important, be able to explain the reasons for behaving in a particular way, and perhaps most significantly, to be able to predict how the athlete will act under a variety of circumstances. The more reliable our predictions, the more control we exert over the situation. Developing an awareness of the athlete's perception of self is a way of achieving such an understanding. A workable definition of self is: the system of concepts available to an individual in attempting to define him or herself.

A person tends to continually construct and re-construct notions, ideas and images about themselves through their experiences in dealing with the events around them. Thus at one point an individual may construe themself as volatile and at other times as quite calm, or as perhaps aggressive when competing but sensitive when outside competition. However in spite of such vacillations, there is generally a core and stable sense of self which persists through experience. Thus a person might see themself as genuine despite at times being both aggressive and sensitive. This conception of self provides three maxims:

- an understanding of self is achievable through inviting the person to describe himself,
- the self is essentially stable,
- some aspects of self are changeable under different circumstances.

Such a model suggests the 'private' world of the athlete can be made more 'public' to those working alongside him. It also suggests the enhanced understanding will foster a better and improved working relationship between them. Questions over whether to push, encourage, direct, cajole or lay off the athlete become more comprehensible, in addition to being able to foresee how the athlete might react in various circumstances. Three aspects of self are worth constructing:

Self image
Self esteem
Self vulnerability

Self image

This can be regarded functionally as the vision the athlete has of himself along axes of discriminations or constructs available to him. The first step is to invite the athlete to describe himself. This might be done by asking him for a description or asking him to select descriptions that best represent the way he sees himself from a list as illustrated in Table 4.1. Between eight and ten descriptions is an optimum number. These descriptions are then written on to a *self awareness* profile as shown in Figure 4.1. The descriptions are as given by the athlete, and should not be altered.

Table 4.1 A list of self descriptions from which the athlete chooses the most important

Self descriptions		
– Optimistic	– Pessimistic	– Cautious
– Co-operative	– Active	– Moody
– Shy	– Confident	– Serious
– Calm	– Adventurous	– Ambitious
– Responsible	– Aggressive	– Disciplined
– Cheerful	– Determined	– Positive
– Generous	– Sociable	– Disorganized
– Humorous	– Modest	– Laid back
– Reliable	– Quiet	– Genuine
– Fiery	– Perfectionist	– Impulsive
– Sensitive	– Self-conscious	– Competent
– Assertive	– Impatient	– Unruffled
– Patient	– Considerate	– Kind
– Forgetful	– Outspoken	– Unsociable
– Unconventional	– Bad tempered	
– Hesitant	– Competitive	
– Excitable	– Critical	
– Enthusiastic	– Easy going	

Self awareness

Contrast	0	1	2	3	4	5	6	7	Description

Score

(hatched)	How I am		Self image
○	Ideal		Self esteem

Figure 4.1 Example of the self awareness profile

The subsequent steps in measuring self image are:

- Write the description in the column on the right-hand side of the profile. (It will take up to twelve descriptions.)
- Clarify with the athlete what each description means to him.

- Find out the 'contrast' to each description and write this, in the athlete's terms, in the appropriate column. Asking the athlete to define the opposite of his description, or to describe someone not like his description are ways of eliciting the contrast. Discovering the contrasts provide the 'axes of discriminations' and helps clarify the athlete's description. Thus 'lazy' as a contrast to 'ambitious' suggests ambition is imbued with effort and industry, whereas 'modesty' as a contrast to 'ambitious' implies the athlete construes ambition in terms of vanity and conceit. The contrast thus enhances the meaning.

Self awareness

Contrast	0	1	2	3	4	5	6	7	Description
Brash							▧○		*Shy*
Lazy							▧	○	*Energetic*
Pessimistic					▧		○		*Cheerful*
Can't be trusted								▧○	*Reliable*
Not bothered								▧○	*Determined*
Critical						○		▧	*Easy going*
Frivolous							▧○		*Serious*
No control							▧	○	*Disciplined*
Unfriendly					▧	○			*Sociable*
Cocky								▧○	*Modest*
Not moody				○			▧		*Bad tempered*

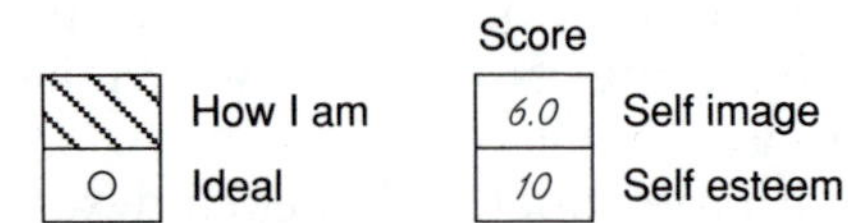

Figure 4.2 Completed self awareness profile

- Invite the athlete to rate 'how I am' on each description, using a 0–7 scale where '7' would be very like the description. This rating is then shaded in on the profile, as in Figure 4.2 and provides a visual display of how the athlete sees himself.
- Calculate a self image score which is the addition of each rating divided by the number of descriptions. In the example of Figure 4.2, this is a score of 66 divided by 11 descriptions giving an average of 6.0.

The ratings of self image can be analysed in a number of ways and will be illustrated with reference to the athlete depicted in Figure 4.2:

- Self image score: this provides an indication of how closely the athlete's ratings correspond to his descriptions of himself. As in Figure 4.2 this score should be reasonably high otherwise it suggests the athlete is not providing very accurate self descriptions.
- Fundamental descriptions of self: those descriptions scored at maximum. This athlete sees himself as reliable, determined, easy going and modest.
- A flavour of how the athlete sees himself: This athlete appears to be self conscious (not brash or cocky) and easy going in his relationships with others but somewhat unfriendly which might be a perception resulting from his cautiousness or from a feeling that socializing will be counterproductive to his sporting needs. Interestingly he also sees himself as somewhat bad tempered. On characteristics which might be considered beneficial in the sporting context – determined, disciplined, reliable, energetic – the athlete rates himself highly.

'When you play tennis you're really exposing your whole soul.'
John McEnroe

Self esteem

This might be defined as the evaluation of self with respect to an idealized vision of self. A measure of self esteem can be made by asking the athlete to provide a rating of 'how I'd like to be' (the ideal) on each of the self descriptions and marking this on the self awareness profile as in Figure 4.2. The discrepancy between ratings of 'how I am' and the ideal, gives an assessment of self esteem. Again with reference to Figure 4.2, self esteem can be analysed in a number of ways:

- *Self esteem score.* This is the summation of all differences in ratings between 'how I am' and the ideal. In Figure 4.2, there is a difference of 1 on 'energetic', 2 on 'cheerful', 2 on 'easy going' and so forth, the summation of the total differences being 10. A high total score suggests *low* self esteem as the athlete construes a big difference between how he is and how he would like to be. A low total score suggests *high* self esteem as the athlete is in effect saying he is close to how he would wish to be.
- *The direction of change.* Usually the ideal is perceived to be close to the description end, as with 'energetic', 'cheerful' and 'disciplined', indicating this is how the athlete would like to be. However, as with 'easy going' and 'bad tempered', the ideal is seen as closer to the contrast end. This does not suggest a need to be like the contrast but to develop a more moderate view of self in these areas.

Armed with such information the athlete can be helped to develop self esteem in those areas presently perceived to be discrepant with the ideal. This will involve:

- Helping the athlete to select one description to work on at a time, which may not necessarily be the one with the largest discrepancy between 'how I am' and the ideal.
- Discussing how the perceived ideal will enhance performance. One way of achieving this is to invite the athlete to describe the advantages of being like the ideal.
- Working through the possibilities for change. This might involve encouraging the athlete to:
  - describe what he would be like and how he would behave if he was one rating closer to the ideal,
  - analyse what he needs to change and what is under his control in achieving the ideal,
  - discuss when he is most like the ideal, and how he may establish more consistency in being like this.

- Agreeing to work on adopting a strategy to accomplish the ideal, and regularly monitoring the progress.

'A man cannot be comfortable without his own approval.'
Mark Twain

Self vulnerability

This can be defined as the conceptualization of self under stress. It is an invaluable way of understanding the athlete's behaviour and attitude when, as they say, 'the going gets tough'. The self descriptions elicited from the self awareness profile are transferred to the central column of Figure 4.3. The athlete is then invited to describe both when he is least like,

Self vulnerability

Least	Descriptions	Most
________	________	________
________	________	________
________	________	________
________	________	________
________	________	________
________	________	________
________	________	________
________	________	________
________	________	________
________	________	________

Figure 4.3 Means of assessing self under stressful conditions

Self vulnerability

Least	Descriptions	Most
After losing, for a couple of days	Ambitious	Spurred on after losing
After a champioship-relax, let the diet go	Disciplined	When I've an aim, such as the championships
When meeting someone for the first time	Easy Going	When around people for a long time
Money problems at home	Assertive	After a good win
When I have trouble making the weight	Enthusiastic	When family doing well
Family arguments	Calm	Relaxing at home
When the weight is a problem	Confident	When I'm preparing well and fit

Figure 4.4 Complete assessment of self vulnerability

and most like the description. Figure 4.4. provides an example taken with an athlete in preparation for a major championship. This type of questioning provides a clear account of what the coach and athlete should both seek to avoid (where possible) and try to ensure happens if the athlete is to perform with self confidence and free from distraction. The profile can be analysed by looking for themes in the athlete's responses. Taking the athlete depicted in Figure 4.4 the themes appear to be:

- *The need for harmony at home.* Disharmony leads to less assertiveness and calmness, whilst harmony gives the athlete enthusiasm and peace of mind.
- *Weight control.* Problems with weight lead to less enthusiasm and less confidence.
- *Previous performance.* Winning increases assertiveness whilst losing initially reduces ambition but then increases it.
- *Preparation.* An aim increases discipline and with preparation going well, confidence increases.

Developing an awareness of how the athlete construes himself is often thought to occur more as a by-product of the coach spending time training with the athlete and observing his reactions in different situations. Understanding the athlete's conception of self can however be achieved by inviting him to make comments about himself. In the sporting context the aspects of self which assume most importance are the image the athlete has of himself, his self esteem and how he is affected by stressful situations. The coach who understands these aspects can play an increasingly significant role in assisting the athlete to perform at his best. In addition, exploring these aspects of self which invite the athlete's participation, can also enhance his own understanding of self.

> 'Boxing gave him his one positive means of self expression. Outside the ring he was an inaudible and almost invisible personality. Inside, he became astonishingly positive and self assured.'
>
> *Hugh McIlvanney* on Johnny Owen

5 Desire

'If you really want something you can get it. Your body will follow your mind.'

Justin Fashanu

The desire or commitment to succeed typifies many successful performances. In psychological terms it might be described as a willingness to risk elaboration into what is, at the moment of risk, the unknown. This demands some explanation. Willingness implies it is a decision, choice or preparedness to commit yourself, and by inference a lack of commitment can also be understood in terms of the athlete's choice. To risk elaboration suggests the decision commits the athlete not just to perform maximally but it also exposes the athlete to self analysis. To triumph means the athlete may have to re-evaluate the way he sees himself and cope with the trappings of success. To fail may mean the athlete being faced with humiliation and a re-assessment of his capabilities and self image. To fail without committing himself does not force the athlete to re-evaluate as nothing was ever put on the line. The final part of the definition – into the unknown – suggests the athlete who commits himself is establishing new boundaries and as such can never be quite sure of the outcome.

Helping the athlete acquire or develop commitment involves the elaboration of three questions:

- What is it he wants to accomplish?
- How badly does he want it?
- What is he prepared to do to achieve it?

The desired accomplishment

It is axiomatic to suggest that athletes endeavour to perform their best for different reasons. A reason, intention, motive, purpose or whatever it is deemed to be called, is from the athlete's perspective, the anticipated gain. Psychologically, what the athlete seeks to gain by performing well has been categorized as: a sense of achievement or mastery, or a sense of approval, recognition or affiliation.

- Achievement or mastery:

> 'There is a need to feel our bodies have a skill and energy of their own.'
>
> *Roger Bannister*

What athletes may seek to achieve includes:
- mastery, perfection;
- a certain standard, criteria or quality;
- their potential;
- a demonstration of ability;
- a new technique, tactic or manoeuvre.

- Affiliation or approval:

> 'There is the desire to find in sport a companionship with kindred people.'
>
> *Roger Bannister*

In this category what athletes may seek is:

- the approval of friends, family, team mates, coach, the press;
- integration within the team;
- recognition amongst competitors and the public;
- honour for the team, club, locality, nation;
- respect.

This list is by no means exclusive. Eugune Gauron (1984) describes nineteen different types of 'motivator' with ninety-five examples. The likelihood is that an athlete will show some consistency in the anticipated gain between performances, so that what 'motivates' him to perform well on one occasion will, in all probability, influence his performance on other occasions. An understanding of what the athlete strives to accomplish will enhance the coach's ability to support him in achieving it. The following open questions crystalize what the important 'motivators' are for the athlete:

1) What three things do you wish to accomplish by your next performance?
   i) ______________________________
   ii) ______________________________
   iii) ______________________________

2) Why are these important to you?
   i) ______________________________
   ii) ______________________________
   iii) ______________________________

In striving for achievement or affiliation the athlete is making a statement about himself – he is seeking to validate some aspect of the way he sees himself. To acquire feedback to confirm, for example, the athlete's view that he is in control, assertive, perfectionist, gifted (with achievement) or well liked, sociable and supportive (with affiliation). This suggests a poor performance puts the athlete, as it were, at risk. It may invalidate some notions the athlete has about himself, and as such he is placed in a position of threat whereby he may need to review the way he sees himself. This can itself be a powerful motivator, as individuals will actively seek to avoid having to reconstrue the way they see themselves.

Poor performances lead to different experiences dependent upon whether the athlete seeks achievement or affiliation. Those who seek achievement or mastery experience guilt if they underperform. They see themselves as letting themselves down, performing below what they would have predicted or expected of themselves. In contrast, athletes who seek affiliation or approval experience humiliation if they underperform. They feel they have let others down or let themselves down in other's eyes. Avoidance of guilt or humiliation are therefore important influences and again become crucial for the coach to grasp in trying to understand how to get the athlete to perform at his best. A third question thus arises in discovering what the important 'motivators' for the athlete are:

3) What three things do you wish to avoid by your next performance?
   i) ______________________________
   ii) ______________________________
   iii) ______________________________

The athlete may need some help to answer this as he may never have considered such factors as important in determining his commitment to perform. Such help might take the form of asking if avoidance of criticism (by self and by others) is important. Knowledge of what are important influences provides the coach with more specific, relevant and effective cues to stimulate the athlete's performance. Table 5.1 provides an example of prompts derived from this model that the coach might employ.

The desired effort

> 'The burning question is how badly do you want to succeed?'
> *Geoff Boycott*

This is the decision to elaborate, to prepare to put yourself to the test, to enter the unknown in pursuit of accomplishing your needs, to risk winning, to go for it. It contrasts sharply with the 'assumed' safety of playing not to lose. As before the athlete may be encouraged to explore what blocks, obstacles and self constraints are imposed to limit performance by considering the following questions:

1) What disadvantages might there be in going all out to achieve what you want?

Table 5.1

	Achievement	*Affiliation*
Wish to accomplish	'Prove it yourself.'	This is for your family.'
Wish to avoid	'Don't sell yourself short.'	'Don't give them the chance.'

i) ______________________________
ii) ______________________________
iii) ______________________________

2) What advantages are there in playing not to lose?
   i) ______________________________
   ii) ______________________________
   iii) ______________________________

Some examples of blocks and limitations athletes may construct for themselves which serve to reduce commitment are:

- improvements becoming increasingly harder to achieve,
- a ceiling to what can be achieved,
- an expectation to perform outstandingly every time,
- an anticipation of feeling uncomfortable with success,
- uncertainty in how to react and cope with success.

The courage to commit yourself to compete without limitations is the mark of a top performer. As Daley Thompson once remarked, 'The only limitations are mental. You can do anything you want, and the guy who thinks positively will win.'

An interesting exercise is **'Go for it'**. This invites the athlete to consider how acceptable the following possibilities are. Those statements having the most appeal can be recorded in writing and kept by the athlete to act as a cue:

G **give** myself *permission* to:
- be as good as possible,
- put in the performance I am capable of,
- extend the limits of my potential,
- go beyond what I've done before,
- enjoy myself,
- make mistakes and learn from them,
- play in a relaxed way,
- be pleased with my progress.

O **opportunity** to *project* myself:
- a chance to present myself in the way I wish,
- an occasion to demonstrate my talent,
- the moment of truth.

F **focus** on *performance*:
- get the performance right and the result will look after itself,
- it's what I do that counts.

O **options** present *choices*:
- be alert for possibilities to take advantage,
- maximize all chances.

R **re-frame** limitations as *frontiers*:
- limitations are self imposed,
- if I choose to put limitations there, I can choose to remove them,
- limitations are frontiers, and frontiers are there to be pushed back.

I **inspire** the *performance*:
- I can picture myself performing as I want to.

T **take** the *risk* of winning:
- all decisions involve risk, because the outcome is unknown. The question is, how badly do I want it?

The desire to make it happen

'He allows himself to explore the extreme limits of his talents rather than settling for a safe mediocrity.'

Vic Marks on Ian Botham

A central tenet of encouraging the athlete to operate with desire and commitment is the creation of appropriate conditions for training and competing. Tara Scanlan and colleagues (1993) have proposed five factors as important in a theoretical model of commitment. They suggest commitment is likely to be greater where the athlete perceives:

- Enjoyment – the need for variety; fun; praise from colleagues and coaches; the athlete given responsibility;

when the athlete is given a specific role to play; when a game plan is discussed; when the athlete's abilities are recognized, utilized and integrated into an overall plan.
- No distractions – the athlete can commit his full attention to the task at hand.
- Personal investment is acknowledged – the resources the athlete invests (time, effort, finance); the sacrifices made (missing time with friends and family).
- Social constraints – where the athlete feels a responsibility to others.
- Opportunities to excel – the chance of mastery; to be able to push the limits back; to find and tap in to reserves; to make things happen.

Promoting commitment to training and performances which extends the athlete's capabilities is a task involving an increase of awareness on the athlete's behalf and an increase in understanding on the coach's behalf. It entails an exploration of those factors the athlete is seeking to accomplish by his performance and those factors he is striving to avoid. Armed with such knowledge the coach is well equipped to assist the athlete achieve. Acknowledging and removing self imposed limitations enables the athlete to push the boundaries back and 'GO FOR IT'. Finally creating the right conditions will enhance the athlete's commitment to his chosen task. Bob Dwyer, the Wallabies coach, made an astute observation on the topic of desire: 'You can't play sport hoping not to lose; you've got to play with an unapologetic commitment to win.'

6 Resourcefulness

'The prizes in life come to those who persevere despite set-backs and disappointments.'

Bryce Courtney

The array of eventualities which might face the athlete during preparation and competition is vast. They can completely knock the athlete out of his stride or, at the very least, create distraction and doubt. The athlete who recognizes the possibility of unpredictable events, prepares in advance to cope with whatever he might be presented with, and is able to dig in when things go against him, is placing himself in an advantageous position.

Possible eventualities include:

- unfavourable playing conditions,
- unfavourable living conditions;
- decisions going against you,
- the odds not in your favour,
- meeting opponents with difficult or unusual styles or behaviour,
- falling behind,
- the final effort,
- overcoming fatigue,
- coping with injury.

'Difficulties are things that show what men are.'

Thomas Higginson

Use the conditions

Figure 6.1 presents a way of analysing and preparing for difficult conditions. A list of competitive conditions is given and for each condition the individual athlete is asked to consider: the most challenging possibility; the best way of preparing for the eventuality; and how the condition might serve as an advantage.

Use the conditions

Condition	Most challenging	Preparation	Advantage
Draw			
Venue			
Changing room			
Temperature			
Lighting			
Playing surface			
Equipment			
Weather			
Ventilation			
Noise level			
Audience			
Officials			

Figure 6.1 Format for challenging unfavourable conditions

The most challenging possibility

This is a positive phrasing of the most difficult situation the athlete is likely to meet.

Some possibilities are:

- Draw – the outside lane; against the top seed; the first to tee off; losing the toss.
- Venue – indoor; open air; closed in; wide open.
- Changing room – cramped; lacking toilets; privacy; security; smelly.
- Temperature – sweltering; brass monkeys.
- Lighting – inadequate; too bright.
- Playing surface – slippery; no give; artificial; frozen.
- Equipment – sub-standard; old; unfamiliar; forgotten or mislaid a vital piece; broken.
- Weather – humid; snow; downpours, driving winds.
- Ventilation – stuffy; smoky; draughts.
- Noise level – deafening; disruptive; lacking atmosphere.
- Audience – heckling; hostile; critical; chattering; boisterous; fidgety.
- Officials – biased; fussy; meticulous.

The best way of preparing for the eventuality

In the middle column (Figure 6.1), the athlete is encouraged to consider, along with his coach or teams mates, how he might best prepare to meet the challenge. By writing solutions on the chart the athlete is commiting himself to managing the situation more effectively. It shifts the focus from the eventuality being unpredictable and unsolvable to being familiar and surmountable. Some possibilities the athlete might consider in preparing for eventualities include:

- Simulation – trying to create the conditions during training, e.g. acclimatization, role playing punctilious officials, practising in the outside lane.
- Visualization – attempting to picture yourself in the situation and coping with it successfully.
- Developing strategies – perhaps best addressed within a group, athletes are invited to discuss and agree on the most favourable responses to 'what if ...' questions. As an example, answers would be sought to questions like 'what if the equipment gives way?', 'what if the wind

suddenly whips up?' or 'what if there is no water in the changing room?'.

How the condition might serve as an advantage

The final column in Figure 6.1 seeks to build on the athlete's preparation in dealing with difficult conditions by seeking ways of construing the event as positive. A convenient way of acquiring a positive view is to seek ways of completing the sentence 'It provides the chance to ...' for each challenging

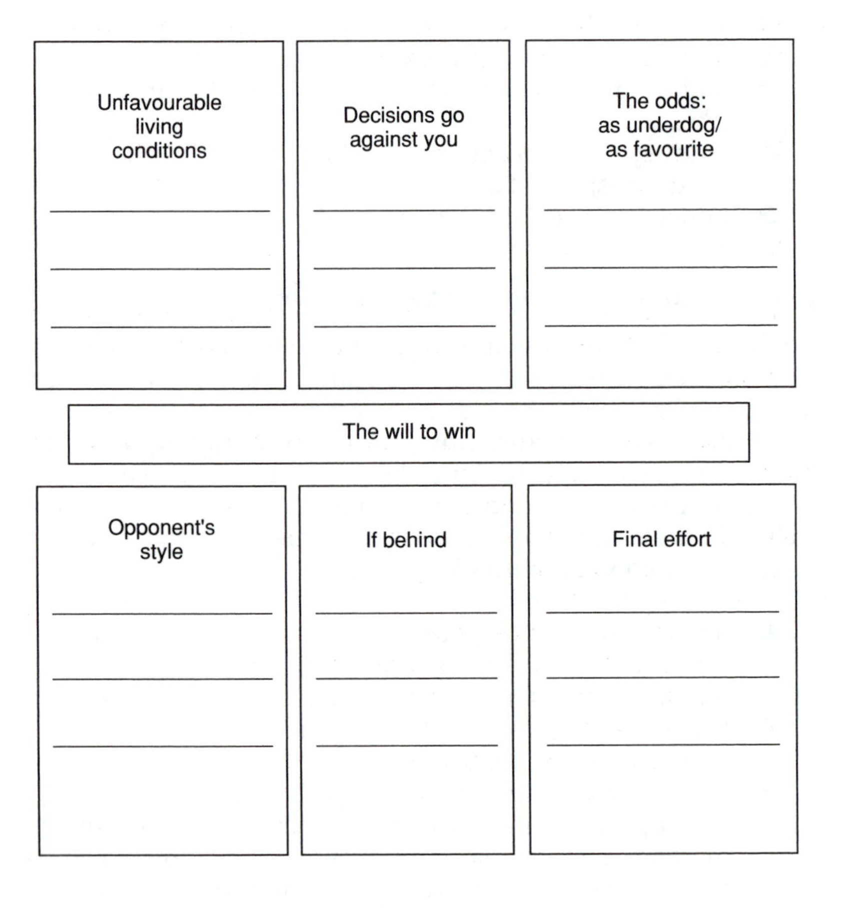

Figure 6.2 'Will to win' chart

condition the athlete is faced with. Brian Lara, the phenomenal run maker, is reported to have responded to a colleague batsman concerned about a seaming ball, with the comment 'It provides the chance to look for the gaps in the field.'

The will to win

This popular phrase is employed here to emphasize a commitment to address six further eventualities – unfavourable living conditions; decisions going against you; odds not in your favour; difficult opponent's styles; falling behind; and the final effort. Figure 6.2 is a chart for use in developing a constructive approach to potential setbacks and disruptions. The essential questions for each of the six sections are:

- What are you likely to be faced with?
- What strategies have you used successfully in the past?
- What are the best options available to you now?

Figure 6.3 provides a sample of an athlete's response to this exercise and illustrates his unique way of preparing for such eventualities.

Some examples of eventualities that might need to be addressed are:

- Unfavourable living conditions:
  - overcrowding, sharing space;
  - long travel, jet lag;
  - boredom, homesickness;
  - unusual diet, drinking water;
  - unfamiliar surroundings.
- Decisions go against you:
  - dubious calls against you;
  - 'legitimate' scores are disallowed;
  - receive a warning, booking, sin bin, standing count.
- The odds not in your favour:
  - as underdog;
  - as favourite.

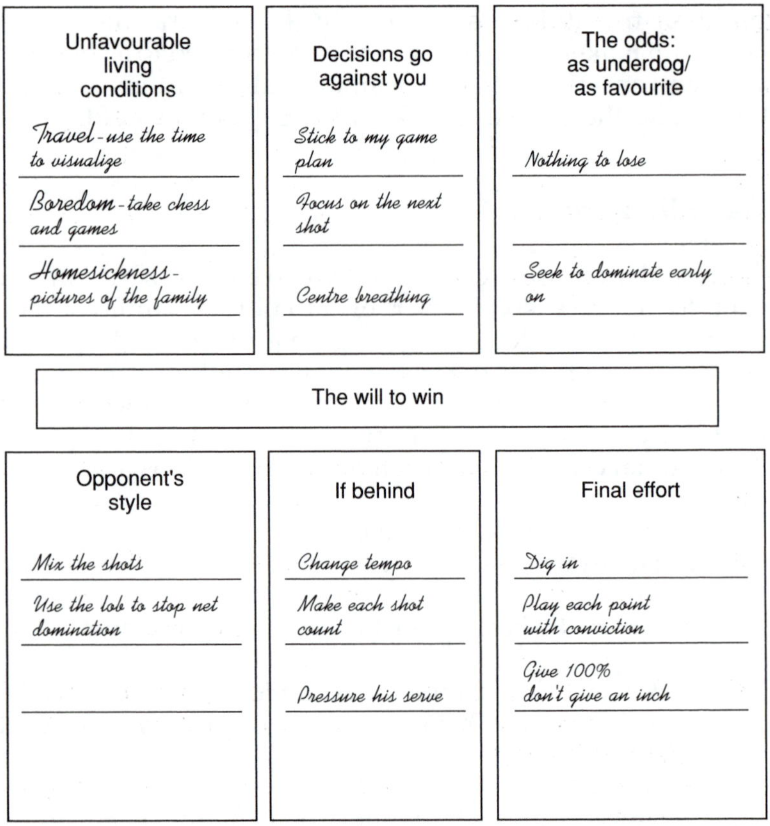

Unfavourable living conditions	Decisions go against you	The odds: as underdog/ as favourite
Travel - use the time to visualize	*Stick to my game plan*	*Nothing to lose*
Boredom - take chess and games	*Focus on the next shot*	
Homesickness - pictures of the family	*Centre breathing*	*Seek to dominate early on*

The will to win

Opponent's style	If behind	Final effort
Mix the shots	*Change tempo*	*Dig in*
Use the lob to stop net domination	*Make each shot count*	*Play each point with conviction*
	Pressure his serve	*Give 100% don't give an inch*

Figure 6.3 Tennis player's completed chart

- Opponent's style:
  - possible tactics that might be employed against you;
  - whether the opponent is known or not;
  - likely behaviour or antics.
- If behind:
  - after an early lead;
  - when trailing from the start.
- The final effort:
  - when ahead.

'Don't compose eulogies to yourself when you get ahead, concentrate on staying there.'

Rod Laver

Overcoming fatigue

The signal to slow down or ease up is usually a psychological one. Thoughts about easing up generally surface before there is a physiological need to ease up. Therefore the initial signs of *fatigue*, *tiredness* and *pain* can be used constructively as indicators or cues to trigger pre-determined actions. Such responses can be practised during selected training sessions when the athlete is pushed to the limit.

> 'What is pain or discomfort to a relatively inexperienced runner, is merely information to the elite runner.'
>
> *Marti Liquori* (athlete)

Fatigue, tiredness and pain can become triggers for the following:

- a commitment to *use your reserves*, empty the tank, go for broke. It is a matter of accessing the untapped physiological capacity. Perhaps time to increase effort, push yourself to the limit, to give it all.
- to *monitor* the feeling. David Hemery (1991) suggests pain can be effectively managed by scanning the body in the following way:
  - become aware of what part of the body is sending the signal,
  - rate the discomfort on a 0–10 scale,
  - judge what rating it would have to be to actually cause you to slow down,
  - keep rating the discomfort and check if it is approaching the limit.

> 'My game has always been to stay until I die.'
>
> *Jimmy Connors*

Dealing with injury

A final and special aspect of resourcefulness is the ability to cope effectively with injury, the curse of the modern athlete at all levels. The inevitability of injury must be recognized. Few athletes make it through a season without experiencing illness or injury in some form. For many it is the worst thing that they perceive can happen to them. To be out of action for any length of time can be a nightmare. It seems the likelihood of injury increases with the amount and intensity of training and competition.

Many athletes tend to either underplay the injury or play on trying to ignore it. This may be the case where the athlete seeks to avoid:

- a loss in status, e.g. losing a place in the team;
- physical inactivity;
- social alienation, e.g. the banter and repartee of changing rooms, the sharing of success and analysis of failure;
- emotional distress, e.g. many athletes prefer the discomfort of training with an injury to the emotional upheaval which accompanies a forced rest from activity;
- cognitive stress, e.g. the feeling of not being in control.

The denial of injury is, according to Weiss and Troxell (1986), a predominant cause of long-term injury. Thus both athlete and coach need to recognize injury early and set about managing it as effectively as possible. Emotional changes are an early repercussion of injury. Aynsley Smith and colleagues (Smith, Scott and Wiese, 1990) describe the typical emotional effect as:

- frustration from being prevented from engaging in activity, elaborating notions about oneself and having ambitions thwarted;
- despair through loss of activity, participation, purpose and sense of control, coupled with somatic symptoms such as loss of appetite, insomnia and upset stomach;
- anger with a venting of dissatisfaction directed at colleagues, coaches, family and inanimate objects such as equipment.

Having a sense or method of coping with injury encourages athletes to take action before further damage is inflicted. The focus here will be on psychological ways of coping, and clearly this needs to be integrated with both medical treatment and physical rehabilitation. What appears to differentiate athletes who cope with injury from those who fail to deal with it successfully are:

- they put the injury in perspective,
- they adopt an attitude of taking control,
- they work on what is available while other athletes merely complain about their lot.

Parameters of effective coping, fully discussed by Butler (in press), are:

- *Understanding and support.* For the athlete the expression of feelings can prove both difficult and awkward because emotions usually have to be controlled so as not to interfere with performance. However in coping with injury the feelings need voicing and venting. The athlete needs to talk through the despair, the unfortunateness and gain a perspective which can involve viewing injury as an 'occupational hazard'. The challenge then for the athlete is to develop a method of handling it.
- *Involvement and commitment to a rehabilitation programme.* This should involve:
  - an understanding of the injury, treatment and prognosis;
  - a means of monitoring progress with, for example, a diary of recovery or a graph of improvement. The Performance Profile can also prove useful here (Butler, in press), with aspects requiring rehabilitation forming the qualities on the profile.
  - meeting small, realistic and achievable targets back to fitness;
  - a contract which represents a public statement about what the athlete will be expected to achieve;
  - complete involvement of the athlete in the development of plans for recuperation.
- *Stress reduction.* Stress has been found to be counterproductive to the healing process (Smith *et al.*, 1990) and

therefore the incorporation of relaxation strategies (Chapter 11) into the rehabilitation programme can prove beneficial.

- *Activity as soon as possible.* Wiese and Weiss (1987) suggest a simple formula for designing appropriate and acceptable challenges. It is based on establishing an answer to 'who, will do what, by when?' For example it might be determined as follows:

Who?	I
Will do what?	will lift five reps at 7 kg resistance with injured leg
By when?	by next Saturday

- *Working on what is under control.* Physical inactivity provides the athlete with the opportunity to work on aspects of performance enhancement that may, under normal circumstances, not be given due recognition. This might be diet, tactics or visualization. Jane Fleming, the Commonwealth heptathlete, summed this up excellently, 'I've been injured or operated on so many times that I've got my own routine now. First, I'm careful about my nutrition. Secondly, I increase the volume of my mental skills training. Thirdly, I work hard on any rehabilitation exercises that I'm given by the medical staff. Fourthly, I get very specific guidance from them as to what conditioning work I am allowed to do. I've got good trunk strength because I've had so many leg injuries! All in all I look at the factors I can control and then do a good job at controlling them. I think injuries are a good test of an athlete's professionalism and dedication.'

A question emerges. Can injury be predicted? There is accumulating evidence from different sports to suggest that it can. A relationship between stressful life events (occasions which disrupt the athlete's lifestyle) and injury has been repeatedly found. Kerr and Fowler (1988) make two suggestions about the causal link between life events and injury.

First, they suggest life events may hinder concentration, with the athlete being pre-occupied with the events impacting on them, to the extent that they fail to fully attend to crucial environmental cues which leads to mistakes and injury.

The second hypothesis proposes that life stressors exhaust the athlete mentally and physically, and thus fatigue becomes the influential factor, because when tired injury becomes more likely. These two hypotheses are, of course, not mutually exclusive.

The need for vigilance regarding the athlete's level of stress and fatigue is therefore paramount. Early recognition may prevent injury. The method of monitoring feelings, discussed in the next chapter, helps the coach to detect any changes in emotional state. According to Kerr and Fowler (1988) the recognition of fatigue and stress should signal the following:

- reduction in training intensity,
- emphasis on perfecting basic skills,
- stress management (e.g. relaxation),
- discussions about working on solutions to the stresses perceived by the athlete.

7 Monitor feelings

'Pride is holding your head up when everyone around you has theirs bowed. Courage is what makes you do it.'
Bryce Courtney

It seems axiomatic to suggest that the emotional state of the athlete will influence performance both during training and competition. Nevertheless what the athlete is feeling is often the subject of conjecture and assumption for coaches and professionals trying to help the athlete. It is sometimes difficult for athletes to verbalize how they feel because they are generally taught to control emotional reactions as part of competitive preparation and thus will construe emotional expression as foreign to the training culture and environment. Further, some athletes will perceive a show of their feelings as a sign of weakness.

To counteract the problem of verbalizing emotions, a number of scales have been developed which require the athlete to rate their mood. These scales appear less threatening to athletes and therefore provide a means of understanding their emotional experiences somewhat better.

Perhaps the most popular scale is the Profile of Mood States (POMS), a sixty-five-item adjective checklist which measures six facets of emotion – tension, depression, fatigue, confusion, anger and vigour. Morgan (1979) was able to demonstrate that a particular set of scores on the POMS predicted success in Olympic qualification. This has become known as the 'iceberg profile' because it is characterized by low ratings on tension, depression, fatigue, confusion and anger in contrast to high scores on vigour.

More recently, and perhaps more significantly in an applied context, Morgan and his colleagues (Morgan, Brown, Raglin, O'Connor and Ellickson, 1987) have discovered that the POMS is sensitive to emotional changes as the intensity of training varies. The scale thus seems emminently feasible as a means of monitoring overtraining, fatigue and staleness.

Feelings scale

	0	1	2	3	4	5	6	7	8	9	10
Exited											
Confident											
Relaxed											
Quick											
Powerful											
Alert											
Active											
Energetic											
Tired											
Worn out											
Heavy											
Annoyed											
Tense											
Nervous											
Restless											
Worried											
Under pressure											
Dejected											
Embarrassed											
Homesick/ lonely											

Figure 7.1 'Feelings scale'

Efforts have been made to reduce the length of the POMS without losing its sensitivity yet making it quicker to use. Two valid attempts are worthy of note:

- Schacham's (1983) shortened version which contains thirty-seven items covering the original six facets of emotion,
- Grove and Prapavessis's (1992) abbreviated version of forty items which includes five items measuring self esteem in an effort to 'tap a positive dimension of emotion'.

POMS was developed originally for use in the clinical field and despite the adaptations made to utilize it in the sports arena, the sense of measuring psychological disturbance still prevails. Interestingly Grove and Prapaveissis (1992) found the weakest scales in the sporting context to be 'confusion' and 'depression' which are clinically apposite but in a sports setting, broadly irrelevant. The 'feelings scale' (Figure 7.1) has been developed within the sporting context and designed with the following perspectives in mind:

- Speed of administration. The scale consists of twenty items.
- The items, as in the POMS, are adjectives but in contrast to the POMS, have been generated by athletes, not psychologists. They therefore represent more meaningful descriptions of emotional experiences and are consequently more acceptable to the athlete.
- The scale has a balance of 'positive' and 'negative' feelings, thus avoiding an unnecessary and potentially detrimental focus on negative feelings particularly as the scale may be employed throughout preparation for a tournament and close to the competition itself.
- On completion a visual display of the athlete's feelings is produced, enabling the coach to quickly understand the athlete's emotional state.
- The scale has a foundation in psychological theory. The 'feelings scale' is based on a personal construct theory framework, building on the ideas of Mildred McCoy (1977). The theory postulates that emotions arise when

a person's way of understanding events and themselves either undergoes change or is threatened by change. Emotions therefore reflect the person in transition. An elaboration of each item on the 'feelings scale' is provided in Figure 7.2

Excited
An awareness that future events may lead to validation (an anticipation that some aspect of self will be elaborated or confirmed)

Confident, relaxed
An awareness of a goodness of fit of self with the anticipated events (a belief that the individual will match up to the task before them)

Quick, powerful, alert
An awareness of a goodness of fit of self with a preparedness to elaborate self

Active, energetic
A preparedness to actively elaborate (a willingness to risk in order to find out)

Tired, worn out, heavy
An awareness of a lack of preparedness to elaborate self

Annoyed
An invalidation of self construing giving rise to a need to find evidence to counteract the invalidation

Tense, nervous (somatic anxiety)
Restless (behavioural expression of anxiety)
Worried, pressurized (cognitive anxiety)
These aspects of anxiety can be understood as different expressions of an awareness of being confronted by events that are mostly beyond the individual's capacity to construe. It is as if what creates anxiety is not the question of how to perform but rather the question of what will happen should the athlete fail to perform well. It is the implications of failure and the subsequent effect on self construing which is the cause of anxiety, because the answers are too difficult to contemplate.

Dejected
An invalidation of self construing (acting in ways out of character with what the individual would expect of himself) with a sense of helplessness that nothing can be done to change the situation

Embarrassed
An awareness of acting in ways that may alter the way others construe the individual

Homesick
An awareness of a lack or loss of validating events specifically associated with significant relationships

Figure 7.2 'Feelings' – a descriptive analysis using a personal construct framework

The administration of the scale is extremely easy. The athlete is invited to provide a rating on each item according to how he is feeling at the present time. A rating scale from 0 (not at all)

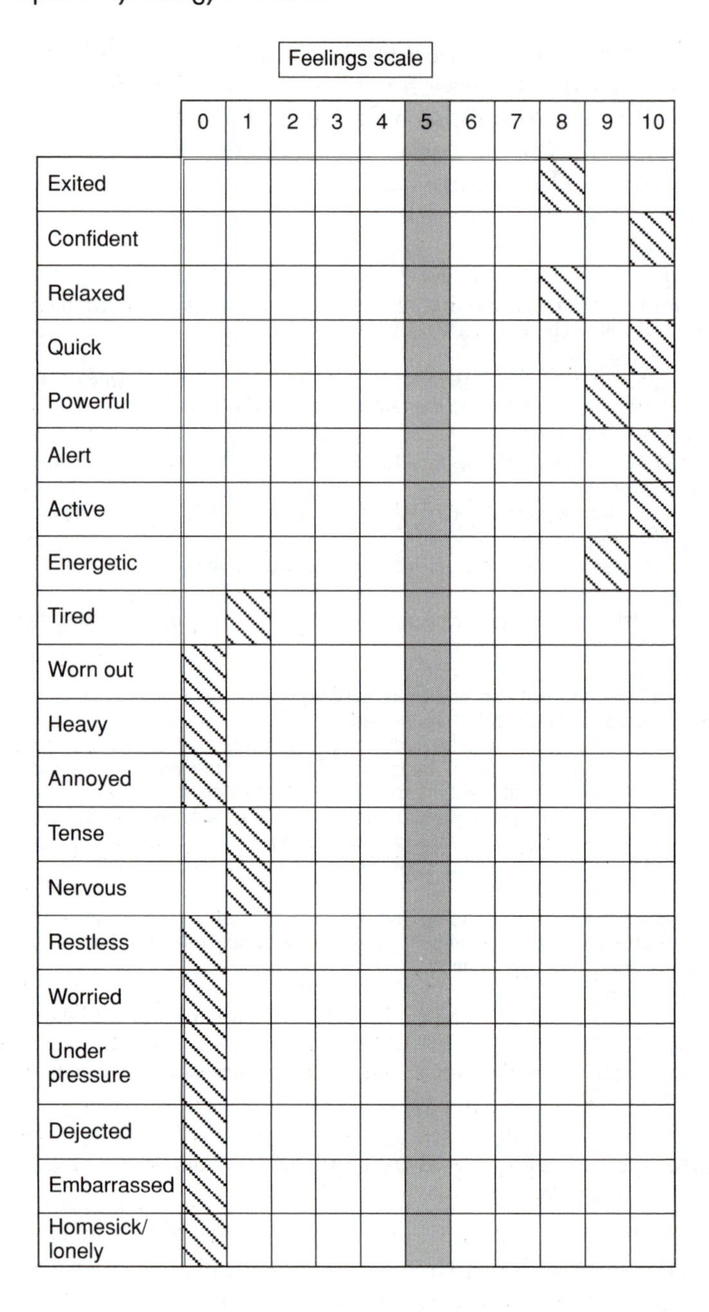

Figure 7.3 Side step profile

to 10 (very much) is used as the measure. The athlete's rating is shaded in the appropriate column as in Figure 7.3 which affords the coach an immediate visual display of the way the athlete is feeling.

Some of the more usual profiles include:

- *The side step profile.* This is, in many ways, the ideal state, illustrated in Figure 7.3, with high ratings on the first eight 'positive' items, contrasting sharply with low ratings on the more 'negative' items. Such a profile suggests the athlete is at an emotional 'peak'.
- *The mazy run profile.* Illustrated in Figure 7.4, this profile can be expected with athletes undergoing a schedule of physical conditioning. It registers the athlete's feeling of being drained of energy. Repeated administrations leading up to the competition and during the taper should see changes in the profile with higher ratings on energy and lower scores on items expressing tiredness, so the profile begins to resemble one more like the 'side step' profile.
- *The mogul profile.* This describes the dips and peaks of a profile that mirrors the skiers' route down the piste. Figure 7.5 shows a typical example which might be obtained during the build up to a competition. The athlete, although feeling generally positive, is experiencing some anxiety in the form of somatic changes (tension and nervousness) coupled with cognitive changes (worry and feeling under pressure).
- *The blip profile.* Occasionally the profile will be distinguished by a single item being rated differently from usual. This might signal a plea for help on the athlete's behalf. It may depict the athlete's annoyance or anger over an issue the coach is not aware of, a sense of dejection or sadness about an event unconnected to the sporting domain, or highlight the emergence of homesickness. Such profiles call for the coach or psychologist to provide a climate for the athlete to discuss the issue, feel understood, and supported in any changes that are made to try and resolve the emotional strain. Hopefully in this way problems can be detected and dealt with

before they interfere dramatically with the athlete's training programme.

- *The collapsed profile.* As illustrated in Figure 7.6 this type of profile immediately signals concern. The athlete is experiencing both fatigue and stress and, as discussed in the last chapter, in this state becomes especially vulnerable to injury. Regular monitoring of athletes with the Feelings Scale should detect minor changes occurring before such a state of stress is reached.

The quick and easy administration of the Feelings Scale, coupled with the useful information it provides on the athlete's emotional experience suggests it can become almost a daily means of monitoring change and progress. Assessment, of course, is only a first step but when furnished with an understanding of the athlete's feelings, the coach or psychologist is much better placed to support the athlete or adapt a training schedule better suited to their needs.

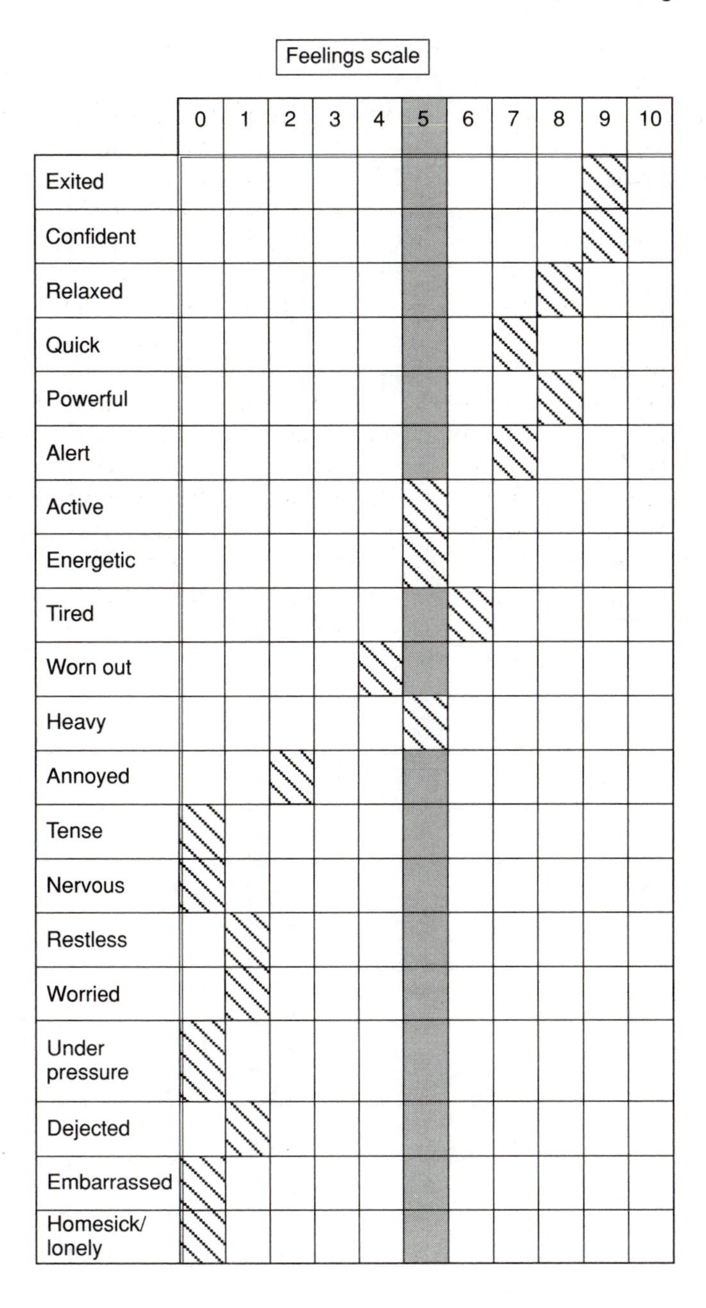

Figure 7.4 Mazy run profile

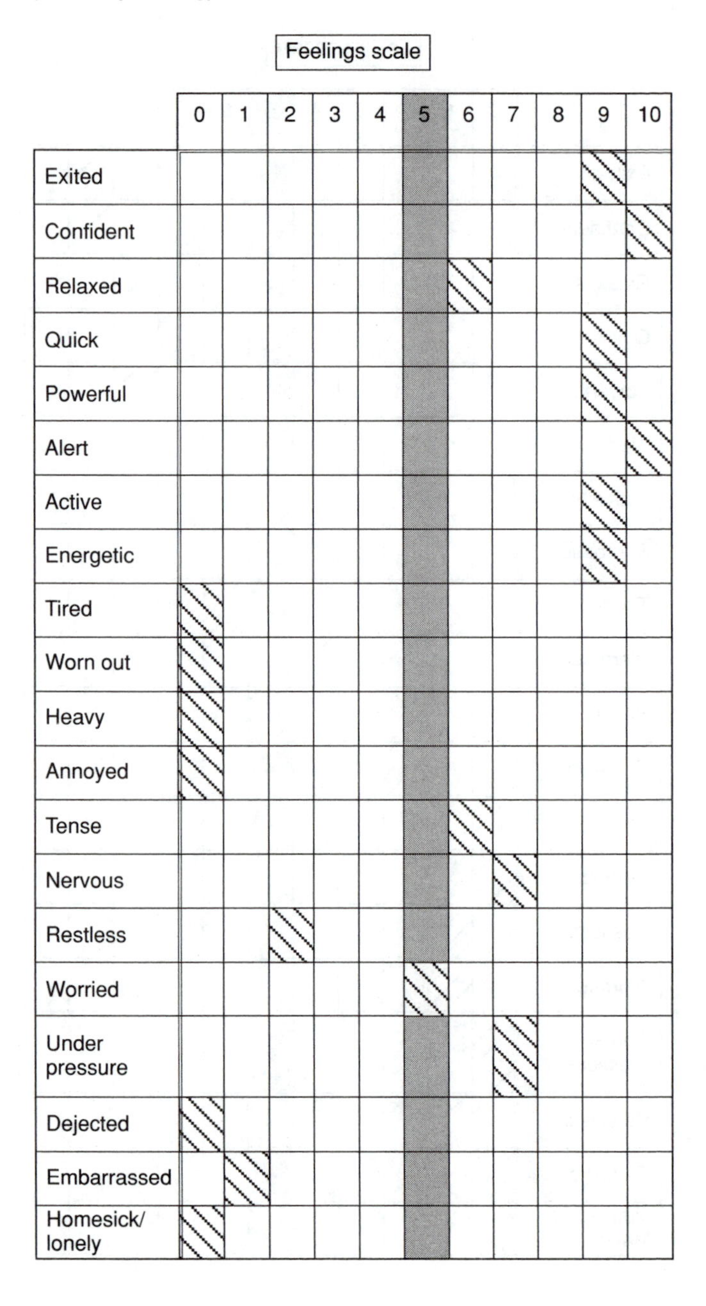

Figure 7.5 Mogul profile

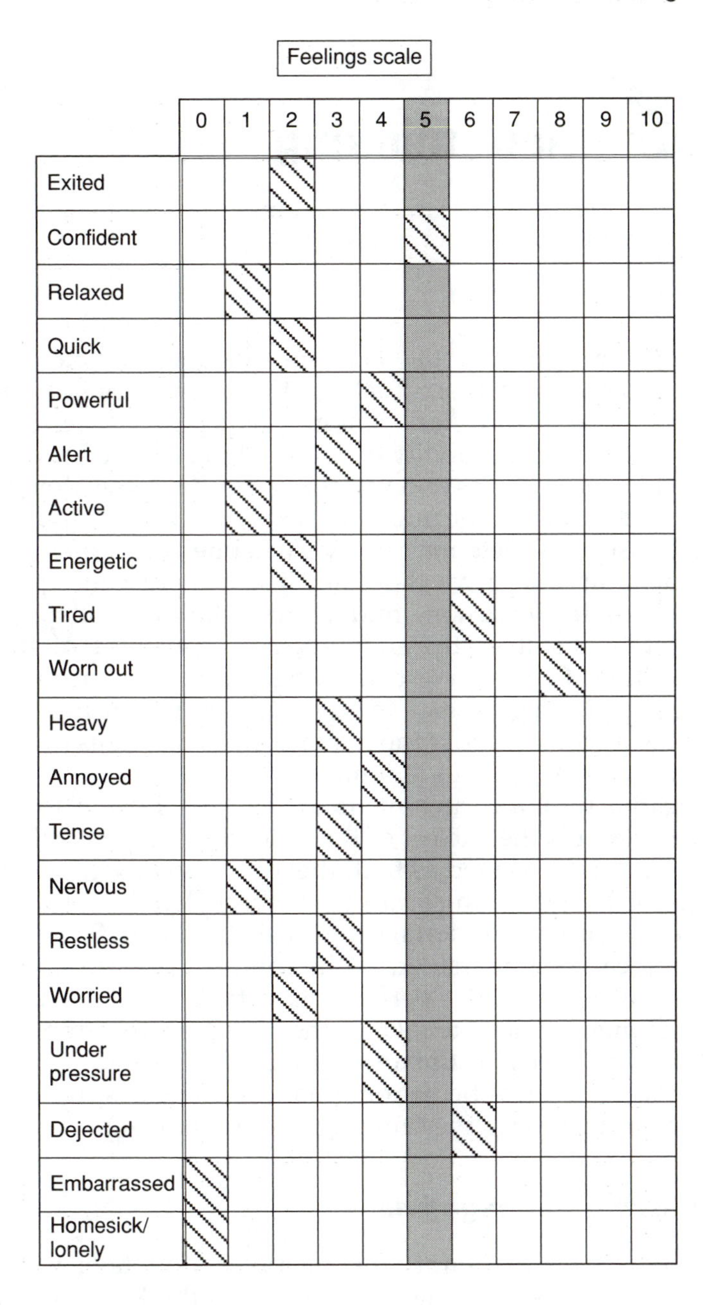

Figure 7.6 Collapsed profile

8 Clear thinking

'The athlete must learn that the mind is something to think with, not just for worrying.'

R. V. Ganslen

One of the items on the Feelings Scale described in the previous chapter is 'worry', a cognitive expression of anxiety. 'Worry' is any form of thinking which undermines the athlete's belief or capability of undertaking a task. Inevitably it can take many forms and varies in severity. A few doubts as the competition nears might be expected but in the more severe case an athlete may be overwhelmed with disruptive, incapacitating, negative thoughts. They might consequently 'freeze' on the occasion, find their technique collapses or completely disintegrates and dread the prospect of future competition. Gordon West, the England and Everton goal-keeper, it is alleged, had to give up his promising career because of worries about the home crowds reactions to any of his errors (O'Hagan and Maume, 1994).

Negative thinking can be construed as the 'flipside' to confidence, which is the subject of the following chapter. Whereas confidence is perceived as both the athlete's conviction about successfully performing a task (self efficacy) and an assurance in their ability to undertake the task (self belief), negative thinking can be understood as the contrast. A lack of conviction about successfully performing a task and/or a lack of belief in their capacity to take on the task. Negative thinking is therefore a 'faulty' estimate of effectiveness and/or ability which leads to an anticipation of failure. Whereas confidence can be built on, negative thinking requires erasing.

Identifying the negatives

The first step is to identify the negatives, doubts or worries. This necessitates listening to the athlete's thinking, achieved usually by asking him to deliberate on the following questions:

- Tell me about your last performance.
- What do you think needs improving or working on?
- What will be your approach to the next performance?
- What might hinder you producing one of your better performances?

The coach might need to listen carefully for hints, cues or key phrases which suggest the presence of negative thinking. He might need to reflect on his own thinking to see if he is transferring any negative thinking in his communication with the athlete. Negative thinking can become so automatic that it requires an 'outside' observer – someone not enmeshed in the training régime – to identify negative patterns. Sometimes athletes will prefer to elaborate on the questions in private and a particularly useful method in such instances is the audiotape where the athlete can record and later replay his responses observing any negatives. When using this method the athlete should always erase the tape after completing the exercise so that it can never become public.

Negative thinking is characterized by seven forms of expression. When listening to the athlete, note the presence of any of the following:

1) *Don'ts.* This includes all 'n'ts' such as 'shouldn't', 'wouldn't' or 'didn't', e.g. 'don't hook the shot'; 'shouldn't tense up when I fall behind'; 'don't pitch it short'.

   Tom Kubistant (1986) makes the point that such statements only serve to introduce the idea of what *not* to do. It is as if the 'don't' is ignored and the main body of the statement becomes the focus to act on. Thus the athlete focuses on hooking the shot, tensing up when behind or pitching short.
2) *Limitations.* These are self imposed barriers about future performance, expressed as statements often preceeded with 'can't', 'never' or 'doubt', e.g. 'I can't hope to get a personal best today'; 'I've never competed well at this venue'; 'I doubt my programme will score well'. Limitations, of course, define what is expected of the athlete and fail to challenge what is possible.

3) *Put downs.* These are statements relating to the athlete's perceived weaknesses or errors in a previous performance, e.g. 'my backhand was weak'; 'I started too slowly'; 'I mis-timed too many tackles'; 'I hit the first hurdle again'. Put downs can come to dominate the athlete's thinking, overshadowing the strengths and pluses in the performance. They may also become self fulfilling. When an athlete thinks of himself in a particular way he may either:
   - expect to act in this way (e.g starting slowly) and thus reinforce this view of himself, or
   - consciously or subtly try to avoid using the technique (e.g. using the backhand) which confirms the impression of being weak in this aspect.
4) *What ifs.* These describe a negative loop. The worry is phrased in terms of a question to which there appears no answer for the athlete, leading him to repeatedly pose the question to himself, e.g. 'what if I'm not selected?'; 'what if I let the side down?'; 'what if I get boxed in?'
5) *Self doubt.* These are expressions of doubt about having the ability to perform well. They may reflect a concern over physical readiness, technical ability or psychological preparedness, e.g. 'I'm not as fit as I should be'; I'm playing and missing too often'; 'I still get angry when making an unforced error'. This of course can be self fulfilling, becoming the source of information upon which the athlete evaluates himself, so perpetuating the doubt.
6) *Letting others down.* This is a concern about how other people might be perceived to have judged the performance, e.g. 'others will be disappointed'; 'I've shown myself up'; 'the press will slaughter me'; 'I've let my coach down'. Central to this thinking is the fear of humiliation and criticism and an awareness that it may involve a change in how other people think of and relate to the athlete.
7) *Preoccupations.* This refers to non performance related problems such as domestic issues, relationships and employment which invade the athlete's thinking and cause distraction.

The effect of negative thinking

Some of the consequences have already been discussed. In summary they include:

- mis-focusing – attending to errors,
- self fulfilment – performing in the way expected,
- perpetuation of the thinking through reinforcement,
- circular questions,
- playing not to lose – restricting performances to mediocrity and avoiding risk,
- trying to please others rather than focusing on performance,
- becoming tense,
- reduced confidence.

The lack of confidence is well described by John Barnes, 'I've gone through periods when I've thought I'm a bad player. It can be because of just one incident, something in one game where I couldn't control the ball – you miscontrol the ball and you think, shit, that was an easy ball, and all of a sudden it's in your mind, asking why you didn't control it.'

Developing clear thinking

A variety of methods are described below in relation to the seven types of negative thinking.

Don'ts

1) *Re-phrase*
The objective is to avoid statements which describe what is not supposed to happen and supplant them with clear declarations of what the athlete should be focusing on. Encourage the athlete to think 'what I need to do is ...' For example, instead of thinking 'don't hook the shot', the athlete might think what he needs to do is: 'relax shoulders', 'visualize where the ball will go', 'breathe out on the downswing' and 'keep my eye on the ball right through the swing'.

'Concentrate on performance.'

Malcolm Cooper (shooter)

Limitations

2) *Believe in the possible*

'The art of kicking is to believe in the possible.'

Fred Allen and *Terry McClean*

The aim of this exercise is to perceive the performance as a challenge rather than as a routine fraught with obstacles and limitations. It consists of asking the athlete to consider the following questions in relation to the next performance:

- What is the dream performance?
- What is possible?
- What is needed to achieve the possible?

Again this focuses the athlete's thinking on what is required in order to produce an appropriate performance. The third question is, in many respects, a goal setting exercise designed to encourage the athlete to make some performance tasks which take him beyond the self imposed limitations.

This type of thinking is well documented in the case of the American swimmer who dreamt of Olympic gold (the dream). He worked out what time would be needed to win the gold at the next Olympics and by how much he would have to improve his performance to achieve this time (the possible). He then calculated he would have to improve his daily training time by 0.1 second a day (the need). By now viewing it as a challenge he stuck to this schedule and at the next Olympics he did indeed produce a performance good enough to take gold.

3) *Develop a routeplanner*

Peter Terry (1989) suggests mapping out a route to turn barriers into positive challenges. The fundamental questions are:

- What stands in the way of performing well?
- What has to be done to overcome the barriers?

Terry gives an example of the process with a rugby player who was frequently flattened in the line out, because of his lack of strength and small size. The planned route to overcome these barriers was: to visualize himself as a 'terrier' to restore a positive attitude, to improve his strength by 10 per cent in four weeks, to construe the advantages of smallness with him being fast compared to the others who were big and slow.

4) *Keep a sense of proportion*
This is a method for keeping the outcome in perspective, and diffusing the repercussions that failure is assumed to bring. It involves reflecting on the following questions:

- What's the worst that can happen?
- What's the likelihood of that?
- Rate the likelihood on a 0–10 scale.

> 'I say to myself that the worst thing I can do is lose a tennis match. That's all.'
>
> *Boris Becker*

Put-downs

5) *See it as unstable*
Put-downs do not have to remain permanent or enduring. It is important to develop a view that weaknesses can be improved upon and recent lapses in form are unstable. Having identified a put-down:

- fix it in the past, e.g. 'my backhand *was* weak', rather than 'my backhand is weak';
- perceive future improvements, e.g. 'there's room for improvement in my catching next time out'.

6) *Confront it*
We seem extremely accommodating and ready to accept our own put-downs. The intriguing question is whether we would be so accepting if we heard someone else putting us down in the same way. One way of confronting a put-down is to put up a defence. Imagine your put-downs and limitations were exposed in the columns of a newspaper, and formulate an appropriate response to it.

What ifs

7) *So?*
Prefixing the 'what if' question with 'so, if …' encourages a response, again based on what the athlete can do to enhance his performance. For example the anxiety laden 'what if I'm drawn on the outside?' becomes a problem-solving statement of 'so, if I'm drawn on the outside I will stay with my game plan'.

Self doubts

8) *Flip it over*
Some aspects of self construing and performance may be habitually framed in a negative way, yet it is always possible to reconstrue them to shed a more positive light on the experience. Some examples might serve to illustrate this:

> 'I don't drop players, I make changes.'
>
> *Bill Shankly*

> 'I'm not old. I just was born before a lot of other people.'
>
> *Darrell Evans*

> 'I am an overweight athlete rather than a fat slob.'
>
> *Robbie Coltraine*

> 'I am not a glutton. I am an explorer of food.'
>
> *Archie Moore*

Let others down

9) *Be your own judge*

> 'He goes out there on the cricket square and doesn't give a bugger what the critics are saying. He just gets his head down and bats.'
>
> *Harvey Smith* on Geoff Boycott

There are two principles to address and accept in developing a stance which frees the athlete from concern over how they think they are being judged or evaluated by others:

- it is impossible to control the way others think – they will make their own minds up,
- people will make judgements irrespective of how the athlete performs – however good the athlete is, someone, somewhere will be critical.

Mike McCallum, the boxer, made this point extremely well with his comment, 'In life you realize you cannot please people. You can move heaven and earth and not make some people satisfied. A lot of people even criticize God the creator.' These two maxims suggest the way people judge you is really their concern, not yours. You are the only one who has the 'inside' knowledge to judge you and therefore that is what should count.

> 'We all like to be liked. As far as I'm concerned I know when I've done all I can do and that's more important to me than what others think, because they don't necessarily know. What they think they see isn't necessarily what's happening.'
>
> *Sean Kerly* (hockey)

Preoccupations

10) *Bag it*

This is a way of putting a potential distraction on ice. Pre-competition is the time least conducive to resolving a problem, because the athlete's focus should be on preparation and performance. Two techniques have proved useful in sidelining the problem until after the competition, when it can be addressed properly:

- Have the athlete imagine a picture of the concern, including all the people involved and encourage him to place a frame around it so the worry is enclosed. The picture can then be hung on a wall and removed only after the event for analysis and problem solving.
- Particularly close to an event the athlete can be encouraged to remove the worry by mentally stuffing it in a kit bag and zipping it up and leaving it there to be recovered after the competition.

11) *Humour*
Finally, humour can be a timely way of dispelling negative thinking. The following quotes represent a fitting way to conclude this chapter:

> 'I couldn't pass judgement on no one. I haven't been perfect myself.'
>
> *Sonny Liston*

> 'I'm that wound up, my jaw is tight, my shoulders tense. I must be the only man in the world with clenched hair.'
>
> *Neil Simon*

> 'If at first you don't succeed, try, try again, then quit. No use being a damn fool about it.'
>
> *W. C. Fields*

> 'It's just eleven of us and eleven of them kicking a little white pill about.'
>
> *Paul Gasgoine*, prior to the World Cup semi-final

> 'You can remember me any way you want to. I don't really care to be honest.'
>
> *Jimmy Connors*

9 Self belief

'I always knew I would do it one day. I always believed'
Mike Powell, after breaking the World long jump record

Self belief can be regarded synonymously with confidence. It is the individual's awareness of his ability to undertake a task. This chapter explores two aspects of self belief: feeling confident and developing confidence in others.

Feeling confident

The definition given above, describes self belief as an awareness about the ability to carry out a task successfully. It may

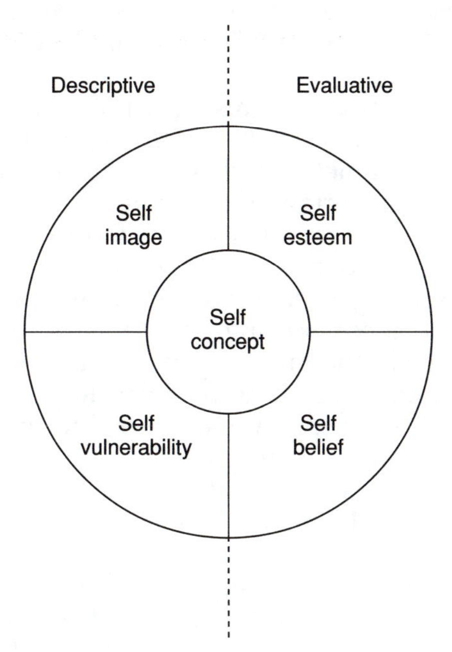

Figure 9.1 Conceptualization of self

thus be conceptualized as an aspect of self awareness, as illustrated in Figure 9.1 which postulates two descriptive and two evaluative facets of self concept. (Self image, self esteem and self vulnerability were described in Chapter 4.)

To summarize:

Self image is the system of characteristics available to an individual in defining himself.
Self esteem is the evaluation of self along the dimensions (characteristics) used to describe self.
Self vulnerability is the perception of change in self occuring under stressful circumstances.
Self belief is the estimate of one's ability to execute a task successfully.

This description of self belief acknowledges the following as important:

- an *estimate* of effectiveness which may range from certainty (highly confident) to uncertainty (lacking in confidence).
- *Ability* which may be present or not. Thus an individual may be just as certain (confident) of *not* having the ability to complete a task successfully as another individual who is certain of his ability.
- Confidence is evaluated in relation to a *task*. This task may be at a 'micro' level so a footballer may be confident of scoring a penalty (the task) by blasting it but not confident about scoring by placing it in the corner. Alternatively the task may be more at a 'macro' level where confidence about a complete performance (e.g. an ice skating programme, a bowling performance or slalom course) is evaluated.
- The *outcome*, defined in terms of whether the athlete will accomplish the task successfully.

Two theoretical models have influenced opinion on the subject of confidence. The least well-known is the 'goodness of fit' model postulated by Mildred McCoy (1977), who, in taking a personal construct perspective, argued that self belief is:

> An awareness of how well a person will match up to the task before them. Where there is a 'goodness of fit' between how the person expects to perform and how they actually perform, then the individual will experience confidence. Where there is a discrepancy between expectation and performance, the person experiences guilt (they have behaved in a way they would not have anticipated of themself). Note this model equally describes a person's lack of confidence in 'goodness of fit' terms as it does a person's sense of confidence.

The second guiding and renowned model is 'self efficacy', formulated by Albert Bandura (1977). He distinguished between an outcome expectancy, described as the person's estimate that a given behaviour will lead to a certain outcome, from an 'efficacy expectation' which he contended was the person's estimate about whether they could successfully execute the behaviour required to produce the outcome. Bandura therfore suggested confidence is:

> An estimate of how effective the person considers they will be in undertaking the task. Expectations of efficacy will determine whether the behaviour will be initiated, how much effort will be expended and how long it will be sustained. Success, it is argued will increase the strength of self efficacy and failure will decrease the estimate of efficacy.

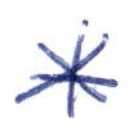

Both the 'goodness of fit' and self efficacy models are combined in Figure 9.2 to provide an integrated model of confidence. Faced with a task, the person first estimates how effective he will be in successfully completing the task. Certainty indicates high self efficacy and reference to the right-hand side of Figure 9.2. Uncertainty about how effective they will be suggests low self efficacy which is presented on the left-hand side of Figure 9.2. The outcome of engaging in the task then influences the individual's self belief. Three processes are postulated:

- The estimate of efficacy is *validated* – high self efficacy is met with success (e.g. the rugby player expects to succeed with a conversion kick and subsequently does so); low self efficacy is met with failure (e.g. the novice skier expects to career out of control first time down the

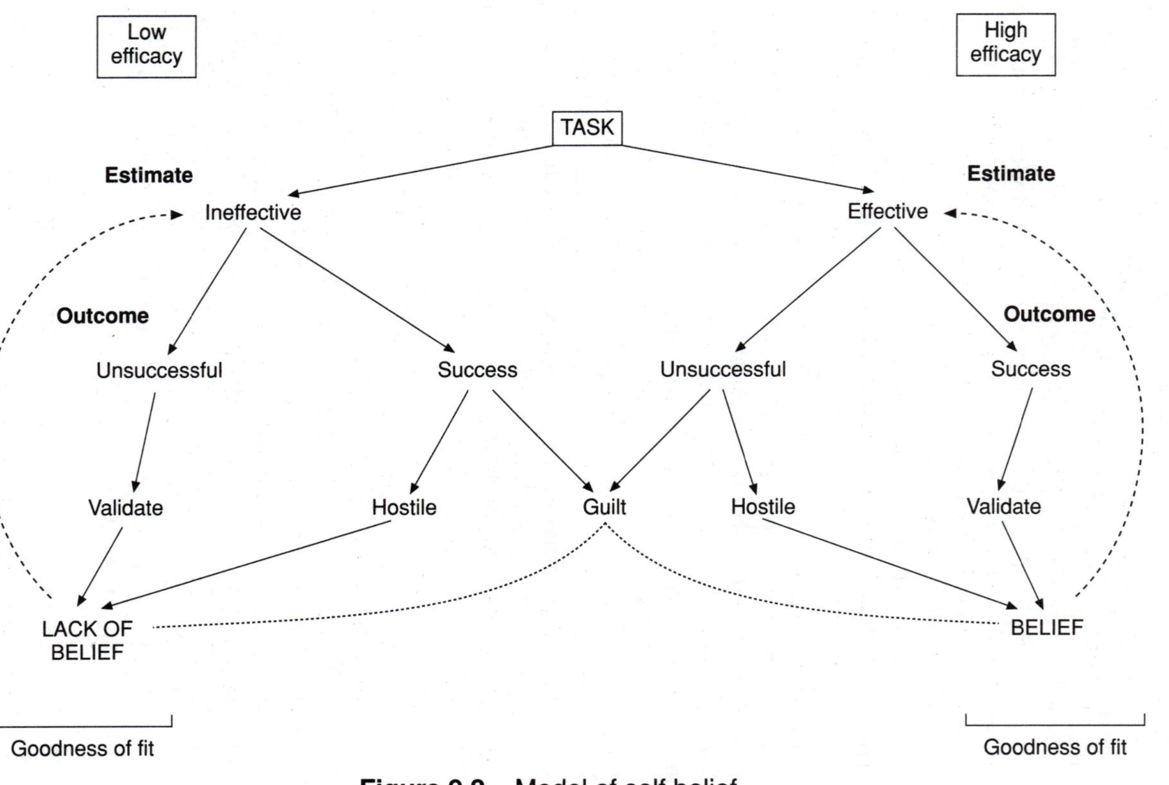

Figure 9.2 Model of self belief

piste and subsequently does just that). Here there is 'goodness of fit' between expectation and outcome resulting in confirmation of ability. This sense of mastery strengthens self belief.

- The estimate of efficacy is *invalidated* leading to *hostility* where the outcome is uncommon. Hostility from a personal construct theory perspective (Bannister and Fransella, 1986) is the individual's effort to protect the view they have of themselves despite evidence to the contrary. It may appear as an effort to tamper with the evidence. There will be a tendency to rationalize, excuse or explain why the performance or outcome was different to what was expected. Thus the archer who scores lower than he expects may put this down to poor conditions, a bad draw or a new piece of equipment. This hostility preserves belief in his ability. On the other hand, the novice golfer who chips a shot to the green which exceeds all his expectations might rationalize it as beginners' luck. This again would be a hostile reaction because it confirms the view that he does not have the ability to perform the shot consistently and thus a lack of belief in his ability is confirmed.
- The estimate of efficacy is *invalidated* leading to *guilt* where the outcome becomes more common. Guilt from a personal construct theory outlook is the individual's recognition of a need to alter the way he views himself. It may appear as surprise following an unexpected outcome. Thus an opening batsman with a run of low scores may feel he has let himself down by performing consistently below his expectation. He may construe it as a loss of form which may consequently lead to a lack of belief in his ability. On the other hand a gymnast who perfects a vault after many previous failed attempts may experience guilt in the form of having to re-evaluate his belief in being able to master the move.

Figure 9.2 suggests the athlete's estimate of efficacy determines how they will approach the task, an estimate fundamentally driven by the athlete's self belief. The coach and psychologist must therefore seek ways of enhancing this estimate, in order for the athlete to feel confident about his performance. The estimate is, according to Albert Bandura (1977), derived from four particular sources of information:

- *Enactive* – the acknowledgement of performance accomplishments, i.e. what the athlete recognizes has been achieved by his participation. Theoretically, this is a durable source of information because it directly influences the athlete's sense of personal mastery (e.g. 'if I've done it before, I can do it again'). Robert Weinberg and colleagues (Weinberg *et al.*, 1979) confirmed the potency of such information by demonstrating that by directing the athlete's focus towards performance accomplishments both efficacy and subsequent performance were enhanced.
- *Vicarious* – the observation that someone of equivalent ability can accomplish the task successfully. Theoretically this source of information is somewhat vulnerable because, as Bandura explains, it is inferred from social comparison (e.g. 'If he can do it, then so can I') and not from personal experience. However Deborah Feltz and colleagues (Feltz, 1982; Feltz and Mugno, 1983) found various forms of modelling (attempting to copy the actions of another person) did improve efficacy and subsequent performance.
- *Exhortative* – verbal persuasion. Bandura suggests this is a weak source of information theoretically because there is no experiential basis for the athlete. Research within the sporting setting also bears this out (Mahoney, 1979).
- *Emotive* –the ability to control arousal levels. It is argued theoretically that increased self efficacy follows performances where the individual effectively manages the physiological state of arousal. This does not however appear to be confirmed by research findings which show effective management of anxiety increases a sense of mastery over arousal control, but not necessarily a consequent increase in self efficacy.

What therefore appears apposite is that strategies aimed at developing the athlete's sense of accomplishment are the most effective means of enhancing self efficacy and subsequent performance. An exercise designed to achieve this is illustrated in Figure 9.3 and called 'a positive frame of mind'. It can be undertaken individually or in groups and invites the athlete to describe three aspects of himself under the headings.

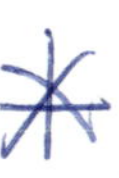

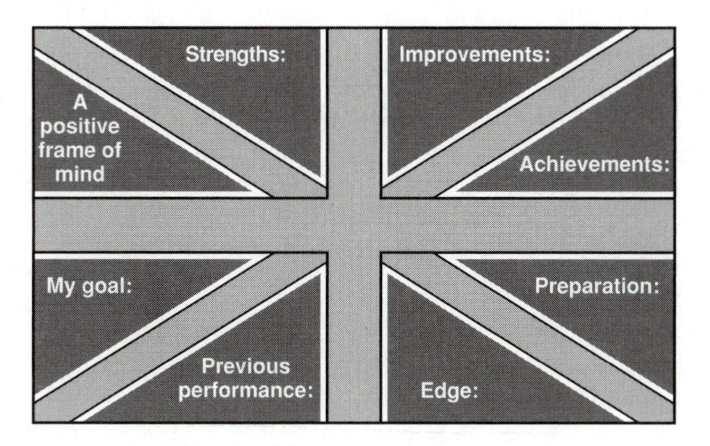

Figure 9.3 Means of enhancing confidence through focusing on performance accomplishments

All descriptions must:

- Be phrased positively.
- Be in the athlete's own words.
- Refer to behaviours the athlete can control. Thus while 'age' might be considered to give the athlete an edge, it is not within his control. Asking the athlete what it is about his age which gives him an edge – e.g. enthusiasm, speed, single mindedness – would provide better statements for him to record.
- Refer to specific events or behaviours rather than global terms like 'personality'. A similar question concerning what it is about his personality – e.g. thoughtful, courageous, assertive – provide more specific and controllable descriptions.
- Be written down on the chart.

The six headings are: strengths, improvements, achievements, preparation, edge and previous performance.

Strengths

> 'An estimation of my own ability is far more important than that of any selector.'
>
> *Stuart Barnes*

Three statements describing what the athlete considers his strengths, attributes or qualities in the sporting context. These may be taken from the performance profile (Chapter 2) where qualities are rated by the athlete. They must be athlete-generated and not provided by the coach or psychologist. As Stuart Barnes implies, it is what the athlete thinks that is important, not what others believe the athlete's assets to be.

Improvements

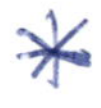

> 'I'm hitting the driver so good, I gotta dial the operator for long distance after I hit it.'
>
> *Lee Trevino*

Three statements describing what the athlete considers he has improved on during the last six months.

Achievements

> 'A silver here gives me every confidence for the Commonwealth Games.'
>
> *Steve Smith*

Three statements outlining accomplishments, successes and realizations which the athlete feels particularly satisfied with.

Preparation

> 'Preparation was the key. I had great sessions during the build-up. My training was organized and planned. I paid attention to detail. I visualized myself winning.'
>
> *Liz McColgan*

Three statements relating to aspects of preparation which have gone well. Liz McColgan mentions four aspects – organized and planned training, attention to detail and visualization.

Edge

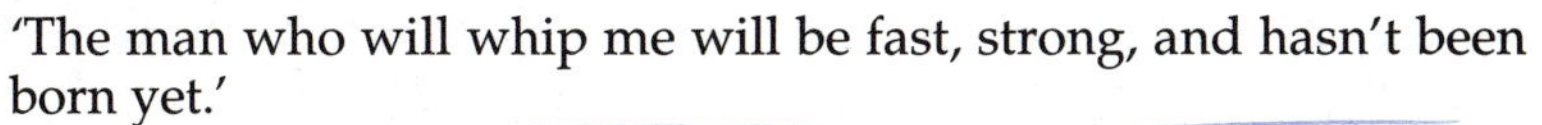

> 'The man who will whip me will be fast, strong, and hasn't been born yet.'
>
> *Mohammed Ali*

Three statements, where possible, of those advantages the athlete perceives he has in comparison to those athletes he will be competing against. In this section it is often difficult for the athlete to find three examples, so one distinct advantage is sufficient.

Previous performance

> 'I've bagged ten wickets each time I've played at Headingley, so I'm looking forward to a repeat in this test.'
>
> *Alan Donald*

Descriptions of three positive aspects of a previous performance. This may be the performance last time out, the last time the athlete competed at the same venue, against the same opponent or at the same stage of the tournament.

'My goal'

The final section of Figure 9.3 is entitled 'My goal', which assists the athlete to focus on what he intends to accomplish during the next performance. (Setting goals was discussed in Chapter 3 and only a bare outline will therefore be given here.) Robert Weinberg (1994) defined a goal simply as 'what an individual is consciously trying to do'. Because effective goals should be *controllable*, *realistic*, *process* – rather than outcome-oriented, and *positively* phrased, a goal for the next performance can be established by completing the sentence: What I aim to do is ...'.

Here 'I' suggests it is something the person has control over; 'aim' implies an achievable but challenging target; and 'to do' directs the athlete to consider the required behaviour, not the outcome.

Athletes use the findings of this exercise in a variety of ways. It is most effectively employed close to a competition when most of the preparation is complete and the athlete is being encouraged to focus on the positive aspects of his forthcoming performance. Some athletes keep the 'Positive frame of mind' in a kit bag or on a prominent wall so they frequently come face to face with self-generated reminders of their accomplishments. Many athletes update the 'frame' following performance so that it remains relevant.

Developing confidence in others

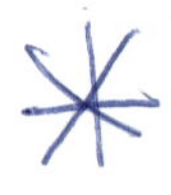

> 'My coach knew I could do it. That gave me the inspiration and confidence to go out and win it.'
>
> *Du'aine Ladejo*

A significant task for the coach, psychologist and other support staff must be to discover ways of improving the athlete's confidence. Given the previous discussion this would seem to centre on encouraging the athlete to focus on his performance accomplishments. Deborah Feltz and colleagues (Feltz and Doyle, 1981; Feltz and Weiss, 1982) and Dan Gould and colleagues (Gould *et al.*, 1989) proposed a series of techniques, which in theory, should serve to enhance the athlete's confidence. However, Gould and colleagues found some techniques were employed relatively scarcely and suggested this might have either been because coaches found them to be ineffective or because coaches were less familiar with their use.

The following techniques can be employed (see Figure 9.4):

- *Praise* – best delivered with emphasis, genuinely directed and immediately following a successful attempt or accomplishment.
- *Feedback* – the immediate relaying of information about a performance, either of an objective nature (e.g.

Developing confidence		
1 *Praise* –Immediate	2 *Feedback* –Immediate –Information (knowledge of results)	3 *Positive statements* –Strengths –Abilities –What he is good at
4 *Work/develop strengths* –Fine tuning	5 *Encourage self statements* –Positive self talk	6 *Verbal persuasion* –Coaxing –'You can do it' type statements
7 *Frame positively* –Not what is not expected –No 'no's	*Focus on performance accomplishments*	8 *Analyse performance* –Highlight successes –Attribute internally (stable)
9 *Encourage reflection* –Athlete's assessment of performance (e.g. rating)	10 *Visualize* –Successful performance –Expected performance	11 *Emphasize advantages* –Edge
12 *Focus on performance, not on outcome* –What the athlete did/ or has done to achieve the successes	13 *Emphasize readiness* –Well prepared –Arousal level	14 *Expect success* –Based on preparation and previous performance

Figure 9.4 Means of enhancing confidence in others

time) or subjectively (e.g. commenting on improved technique).

- *Positive statements* – emphasizing the athlete's qualities and attributes as perceived by the coach, psychologist or support staff.
- *Work on strengths* – the fine tuning of techniques an athlete is particularly adept at.
- *Encourage self statements* – inviting the athlete to remind himself of his strengths and abilities.

- *Verbal persuasion* – coaxing, enticing, persuading the athlete that he is capable and able to perform successfully.
- *Frame positively* – delivering instructions in a way which does not allude to what is not expected (e.g. 'don't stay on the baseline', 'no shuffling across the crease', 'don't hook into the trees' all carry information and an expectation about how the athlete should *not* perform which 'sows the seed of doubt'). All such information can be expressed in a positive way (e.g. 'attack the net', 'foot to the pitch of the ball', 'a five iron straight down the fairway').
- *Analyse performance* – evaluating training and competitive performance in a way which both highlights successes and encourages the athlete to believe they are the result of his ability (a stable attribute) rather than his effort (which is an unstable attribute, i.e. it changes from performance to performance).
- *Encourage reflection* – encouraging the athlete to assess his performance particularly following success.
- *Visualize* – inviting the athlete to picture himself reliving a successful performance or to picture himself accomplishing a forthcoming event.
- *Emphasize advantages* – focusing on the athlete's superiority or perceived edge.
- *Focus on performance* – the behaviour(s) exhibited by the athlete which accounted for the success, not the success itself.
- *Emphasize readiness* – stressing how well the athlete has prepared and emphasizing that any arousal is a signal of the athlete's preparedness to compete.
- *Expect success* – providing an expectation of success because of the athlete's previous successful performances and because 'no stone has been left unturned' in the preparation.

Assessing the techniques coaches use in their encouragement of athletes is often best achieved through observation by:

- having another coach observe, monitor and comment on your actions,

- videoing the way you relate to the athlete,
- ask the athlete what instils confidence in him.

The effective use of such confidence-building techniques is dependent both on the individual athlete – what is helpful to one may be counter productive for another – and the different stages leading up to a performance. A useful exercise to address the latter is illustrated in Figure 9.5. This 'time frame' invites the coach to chart both what he is good at and what he might work to improve (from information gained from other coaches, video or the athlete) at the various stages leading to the competition. In this way not only does the athlete benefit

	What I'm good at	What needs improving
Preparation	• • •	• • •
Taper	• •	• •
Planning for competition	• •	• •
Warm up	• •	• •
Competition	• •	• •

Figure 9.5 Time frame for developing confidence

from a relationship moulded to enhance his confidence but the coach is also engaged dynamically in improving his own self efficacy and thus consequently his confidence in his coaching ability.

10 Stay focused

'The secret of concentration is not to let outside factors register. Be aware of them but keep them outside the mental bubble in which you are operating. Concentration is about channelling your mind into a specific area while directing your energies in one direction.'

Geoff Boycott

Geoff Boycott, a magnificent exponent of maintained focus, summarizes the experience well. He refers to channelling the mind into a specific area. This conjures up a picture of the individual surveying the relevant cues in the environment, whilst simultaneously excluding irrelevent cues or distractions, and funnelling the mind towards a point which will trigger the desired action.

This conceptualization has sympathy with Robert Nideffer (1976) who proposed that attentional style can be described as *broad* or *narrow*. A broad focus describes the way a number or range of cues/stimuli are attended to in arriving at a decision. For example, before playing a shot a golfer will survey the lie of the ball, the distance to the green, the club to use, the wind direction, the hazards (bunkers, trees) and type of shot (all external cues or information) plus previous experience of the hole and confidence in executing the shot adequately (the internal cues or information).

A narrow focus describes the process of 'locking' the mind on to a single stimulus which will *trigger* the desired action or performance. Figure 10.1 outlines diagrammatically the process of focusing. This model emphasizes:

- That focusing is a *pre-performance* activity. It is the means by which an athlete prepares to deliver a desired action – the action itself, being executed almost automatically. This is not to intimate that focusing does not happen during performance. Clearly it does. However for it to be effective it will have been anticipated and prepared for in advance.

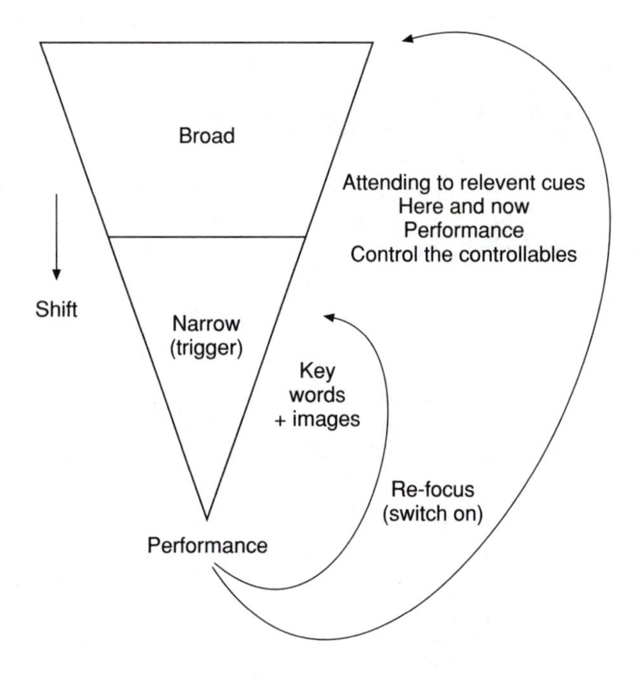

Figure 10.1 The process of focusing

- The need to *shift* focus, from broad to narrow prior to performance. Nideffer (1976) argued that under stress the shift is made more difficult, which may result in an athlete reverting to a predominant, yet not necessarily appropriate, style. Thus an athlete may fail to narrow focus prior to acting or cease to broaden focus during a break in performance when re-focusing is necessary.
- Different performances demand different focusing strategies. Table 10.1 sketches three possibilities linked to different performance demands, categorized as:

  i) *Continuous* performance which necessitates a game plan where actions are triggered by pre-arranged cues, stages or eventualities.
  ii) *Reviewed* performance where 'breaks' in the action

may demand a broad focus to review the situation, prior to re-focusing for the next action.

iii) *Perfected* performance which requires the athlete to follow through a set focusing strategy prior to each performance.

Table 10.1 Types of focusing strategies for different performances

Continuous:		
Skiing	Swimming	Speed skating
Bobsleigh	Rowing	Distance running
Skating	Judo	Short track running
Canoeing	Gymnastics	Cycling
Boxing	Football	Hockey
Rugby	Basketball	
Reviewed:		
Diving	Pitching (baseball)	Free kicks (football)
Golf	Serving (tennis, squash, table tennis, volleyball badminton)	Conversion/penalty (rugby)
Fencing		Penalty corner (hockey)
Bowling (cricket)		
Snooker	Bowls	
Perfected action		
Receiving serve (tennis, squash, volleyball, badminton, table tennis)		Batting/receiving (cricket, baseball)
		Archery
Shooting		Free shot (basketball)
Field events (long jump, high jump, discus, hammer, javelin, shot, triple jump, pole vault)		
Weightlifting		

Developing a focus

Adopting an effective focus requires the athlete and coach to recognize two central tenets:

- Keep thinking in the *now*.
  It is what the athlete has to do at the present moment that counts. Too often the athlete will get caught up lamenting past errors (of the 'if only ...' type),

wallowing in past successes or composing eulogies about the future. Only a focus on the here and now can enable the athlete to direct his performance appropriately.

'Keep focused in the now. It's the only time we have. It's controlling what we do now that determines our progress.'

Kip Keino

- Keep focused on *performance*.
  It is what the athlete has to do that counts. It is sticking to 'racing my race' and not getting caught up with how other competitors are behaving or forecasting future glory.

'People said I was slow off the blocks. I was a metre or two behind, but I started as fast as I could have done. I focused on my race. The others started at a blistering pace but I knew I had started well for me. That was enough.'

Carl Lewis, after breaking the 100m World record, in a race where six men went under 10 seconds.

Developing a game plan

With a continuous performance there are likely to be changes or focus as the performance unfolds. This may lead to the development of a *game plan*, an overview of what the athlete intends to do at each point of the performance. Terry Orlick (1986) suggests a continuous performance can be dissected into stages with each stage having a focus. For example, Orlick describes a 'race focus plan' for a skier which contains four stages – the start (with a focus on warm-up, check bindings, imagery, and explosion from the start); the first few gates (with a focus on explosion, speed and riding a flat ski); the course (with a focus on flow, rhythm, and letting it go); and the finish (with a focus on pushing the last few gates and being strong despite fatigue). A game plan then relies on the athlete recognizing when the stages change (through external and internal cues) and switching to the appropriate focus.

The key to developing an effective *game plan* is:

- identify what you intend to do in order to achieve the performance you want, from the start through to the end;
- associate or tie these proposed actions to 'cues' either in the environment (e.g. the turn in swimming, gates in canoeing, distance in cycling) or within yourself (e.g. fatigue);
- visualize the performance, 'feeling' each cue trigger the desired action;
- keep a written record of cues and desired actions, as in Figure 10.2 which illustrates an 800-m runner's game plan;
- amend following the performance.

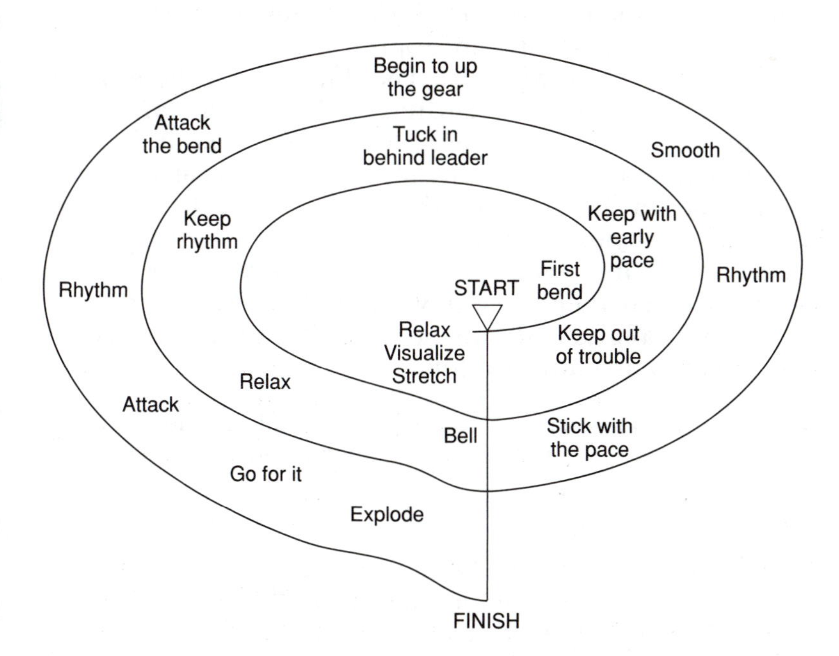

Figure 10.2 Game plan for an 800-m runner

A strategy for re-focusing

In many sports it is not necessary to maintain a focus throughout the event. Those contests which are interspersed with breaks demand the athlete to switch on and off, and as described above can be categorized as reviewed performances. Breaks are typically:

- programmed – half time, end of a set, end of a round;
- dictated by the coach – time-out, substitutions;
- determined by an official – foul, out of play;
- between plays – diving, golf shots, tennis points, snooker shots, shooting, cricket balls, pitching in baseball, field events.

The key is to be able to switch back into focus at the resumption of play. John McEnroe displayed remarkable aptitude for switching back into an appropriate focus following a confrontation with officials. The break is a time to be savoured, to review. It is hardly possible to maintain a high level of concentration over a prolonged time, and it therefore becomes necessary to intensify attentional focus at key times. Sandy Gordon (1990) argues that the most effective focusing strategies are those that minimize the period of optimum concentration. It is being able to switch totally into focus at the key points and then relax, review, and re-focus during the break. Ken Ravizza and Thomas Osborne (1991) describe this as a 'one play at a time' routine.

> 'Although you must look to your concentration, I feel it is also helpful to relax between deliveries. So you learn to switch on and off.'
>
> *Glenn Turner*

In addition to the planned stoppages during a performance there are times when re-focusing is particularly important, times when there may be emotional reactions to overcome:

- after a mistake or error,
- a bad decision going against you,
- if distracted,
- going behind or going ahead.

Re-focusing is best achieved where the athlete has a planned and practised method. The 'switch on' technique offers a routine to follow, one which can be expanded or concentrated to fit the length of the break. As with all techniques it should become part of regular practice during training and amended according to the athlete's needs, wishes and experience.

The basic 'switch on' routine is:

- *Remove* the reaction. Success requires acknowledgement. Errors, doubts and self-recriminations need recognition because they will emphasize the athlete's responsibility to re-focus for the next play. An error might be 'physically' removed by spitting it out, stamping it into the ground, or 'mentally' removed by imagining it being kicked into touch.
- *Recover* through regulating the breathing pattern, relaxation or centring (Chapter 3) which increase oxygen uptake, conserve energy and dissipate tension.
- *Review* what to do next. Reflect on the game plan, making any adjustments necessary. Decide what the next action will be.
- *Visualize* the next action.
- *Cue in* to the event. This might be a verbal signal. Ravizza and Osborne (1991) taught American footballers to use 'ready' prior to each play. It might alternatively be a visual signal, such as the seam of a cricket ball (Bull *et al.*, 1992). Finally it might be a physical signal such as bouncing the ball before serving in tennis.
- *Lock on* to the trigger (see below).
- *Respond.* Trust that your training and preparation has been geared to this moment and action.

'You've got time to think ... you're out there by yourself and you have to think and change things yourself.'

Stefan Edberg

Eliciting triggers

Triggers are words or images which evoke a desired action. They may therefore be employed by the athlete to initiate a regular 'perfected' performance or by a coach in encouraging the athlete to respond in a certain way. The most effective triggers are:

- phrased positively, thus stimulating the desired action,
- short and succinct,
- personal, i.e. elicited by the athlete,
- expressed with conviction,
- practised during training.

There are various ways of eliciting triggers:

A plan checklist

- write a list of words which represents every step involved in the performance you wish to achieve,
- reduce this list to one or two *key words* which best emphasizes what is required,
- practise the key words in training, building it into the performance route.

> 'I used to go through a short plan checklist before shooting. This was a list of words which represented every single step involved in shooting. Then I reduced these to key words so I could go through the list faster. Finally I used one word to emphasize what I wanted, such as "trigger" or "smooth".'
>
> *Linda Thon*

Describe a best performance

- ask the athlete to describe a top performance as if re-living it from start to finish,
- listen for words or statements expressed with conviction, metaphors or vivid images,
- check these out with the athlete to assess how and when they might be used.

Neill Allen, a journalist, once described a performance of Bob Hayes in this way: 'He just exploded, like a clenched fist travelling down the track'. This statement, although not athlete generated, has both a powerful metaphor (exploded) which might be employed as a key word, and a vivid image (clenched fist) which might be used as a key image.

Association

- consider a quality or action which is required for the performance to go well,
- invite the athlete to provide a striking, vivid, dramatic or animated description of what it will be like to complete this successfully. For example:
  - 'as deceptive as a wildcat' (Gale Sayers)
  - 'a pregnant package of coiled venom' (Joe Louis)
  - 'served like a low flying bomber' (Bjorn Borg)
  - 'The grace of a streamlined express' (Jesse Owens)
  - 'Hits like an epileptic pile driver' (Jack Dempsey)

Both key words and key images are effective triggers. The following examples demonstrate how athletes have successfully developed a variety of triggers to help 'lock' on to the desired action or feeling:

> (Technique)
> 'I concentrate only on the ball in relation to the face of my racket, which is a full-time job, since no two balls ever come over the net in the same way.'
>
> *Billie Jean King*

> (Emotion/Mood)
> 'What I try to do is think aggression, think smooth. When I know I've got rhythm I know I'm going to be dangerous.'
>
> *Richard Hadlee*

> (Image)
> 'I imagine a tiger, ready to let loose and sometimes feel myself turning into a tiger.'
>
> *Mark Breland*

> 'I told them to be like cornered tigers, nowhere to go. Just go out and fight.'
>
> *Imran Khan*

> 'In the ring your fists are like snakes that strike before you can tell them to.'
>
> *Sugar Ray Leonard*

11 Arousal control

'Psyched up or psyched out.'

Daniel Gould and *Eileen Udry*

Faced with a situation which is potentially stressful, confrontational or dangerous an individual almost invariably reacts with increased arousal. So much so that the reaction might be construed as universal. The process, which might be almost instantaneous, goes something like this:

- The individual anticipates the possibility of harm, either physically (e.g. pain) or psychologically (e.g. humiliation).
- Physiological changes rapidly occur which prepare the body to face up to the confrontation, including raised heart rate, increased perspiration, increased respiration rate.
- This state is commonly known as a 'fight or flight' response because the physiological changes prepare the individual for action – either by taking on the danger or quickly escaping from it.

Given the potential and perceived 'dangers' of sporting competition it is no surprise that athletes regularly report such feelings prior to competition. The manner in which athletes deal with the increased arousal will inevitably effect the way they perform. Dan Gould and Eileen Udry (1994) have posed three pertinent questions relating to arousal control as a means of assisting athletes to improve their performance:

1) How is the arousal construed by the athlete?
2) What is the relationship between arousal and performance?
3) What techniques enable athletes to regulate arousal levels in order to achieve optimum levels for performance?

How is arousal construed?

Practically, a useful starting point is to ask the athlete to describe what it feels like in the lead-up to a competition. This might be followed by asking about the experience of a difficult or 'high' pressure event. The coach or psychologist should note how the athlete describes arousal as follows:

- What is perceived physiologically (e.g. muscle tension) and what is perceived psychologically (e.g. doubts, worries)? (The psychological components of arousal were covered in Chapter 8.) Where arousal is conceptualized by the athlete in physiological terms, then the arousal control techniques covered in this chapter should prove helpful.
- Is arousal construed positively or negatively? Negative descriptions include experiences like 'nervous', 'tense', 'fearful' whilst positive descriptions include 'pumped up', 'charged up' and 'energetic'. Given that the arousal level is a measure of how hard the body is working in preparing for action, the experience stems from how that arousal is interpreted by the athlete. Similar confrontations or challenges giving rise to physiological arousal will be experienced quite differently by individuals who interpret the event or the arousal in different ways. Thus driving fast may lead to physiological arousal which may be interpreted as exciting or stimulating (leaving the individual feeling good), or panicky and frightening (with consequent dread and fear). In the sporting context it is important to recognize how the athlete interprets pre-competition arousal. Most regard it as a necessary evil. They need to be aroused but interpret the state in a negative way. Perhaps what is important is fostering and reinforcing the belief that arousal is the body's way of preparing for action, and as such is both necessary and a way of signalling the athlete's readiness to compete.
- Is the arousal perceived as localized or general? There are individual differences in where arousal is experienced. Some describe heart rate changes, others muscle tension or stomach churning and yet others sweaty

palms. The 'site' of arousal may determine the method used to assist the athlete in controlling the arousal.

- What terms does the athlete use to describe arousal? For example:
  i) heart rate – palpitations, racing, thumping,
  ii) muscle tension – tense, taught, tight,
  iii) stomach – butterflies, churning, nausea.

  The particular metaphors and descriptions the athlete uses to convey how he is feeling, should be accepted and employed by the coach and psychologist when exploring issues of arousal control.

What is the relationship between arousal and performance?

Much has been written about the relationship between arousal and subsequent performance. Traditionally it is thought that a certain level of arousal is beneficial to performance. Thus warming up and psyching up strategies are regularly employed to raise the level of arousal. Athletes also often recognize that they do not perform well when under aroused or when they do not anticipate a confrontation or challenge. Under estimating the competition leading to lack of arousal often results in below par performances.

Over arousal is also thought to interfere with the athlete's performance. However this relationship is not a simple one. Whilst over arousal is generally recognized as causing deterioration in performance, the rate of deterioration is crucial. Whether the decrease is gradual (and therefore manageable) or catastrophic (and therefore unmanageable) as suggested by Lew Hardy (1990), seems dependent on how the athlete construes the situation. Should the athlete be consumed by doubt (cognitively anxious) the deterioration seems likely to be rapid and irretrievable, but if the athlete shows little cognitive anxiety the deterioration seems likely to be more gradual and redeemable.

The apposite question then focuses on what the optimum level of arousal should be for each individual athlete. Terry Orlick (1986) addresses this by asking athletes to describe differences in arousal levels for two contrasting performances

– a previous poor and a previous good performance. This leads to the identification of an optimum level. The next question relates to what the athlete did to achieve this optimum level, particularly emphasizing what the athlete has control over. Finally, the athlete is invited to consider incorporating such actions consistently into his pre-performance routines so that he can approach each event with an anticipated optimum level of arousal.

- Optimum levels of arousal are not exclusively athlete-determined but are also event-determined. Stuart Biddle (1986) suggests for example, that psyching-up prior to strength tasks enhances performance but does not enhance speed, balance or technique.

Controlling arousal levels

Control is essential. Arriving at an optimum level of arousal demands the ability to regulate arousal levels. This may mean increasing arousal on some occasions and decreasing arousal on others. An athlete who recognizes his optimum level for the task and has the techniques to modify arousal to meet this optimum is clearly enhancing his chances of performing well.

Psyching-up

> 'It means a change in perspective, recognizing that the sensations are signalling that the body is readying itself for fight or flight. Personal bests are created out of that.'
>
> *David Hemery*

Based on Shelton and Mahoney's work (1978) the following mnemonic outlines strategies athletes have successfully employed to enhance arousal levels:

C **cue words:** (words which energize, inspire, vitalize; words which are meaningful for the athlete)
- 'pumped up'
- 'go for it'
- 'seize the chance'
- 'explode'

H **here and now:** (stay in the present; review the controllables, the game plan)
- 'race my race'
- 'explode at the start'
- 'it's what I do that matters'

A **ability:** (review your strengths)
- 'I'm quick'
- 'a chance to improve on what I've done before'
- 'this is my event'

M **mental imagery:** (picture yourself succeeding)
- 'visualize victory'
- 'picture the medal'
- 'claim the rostrum'

P **positive interpretation of arousal**
- 'my body is ready'
- 'I need this energy'
- 'I'm prepared'

Relaxing down

> 'Whatever success I've had is due to being so perfectly relaxed that I can feel my jaw muscles wiggle.'
>
> *Bobby Joe Morrow* (Olympic 100m champion)

Relaxation is best construed as a skill which, like any other skill, may be acquired, developed and mastered through practice. It is a means of achieving control by letting go. This at first seems paradoxical as control is often associated with 'taking a grip' of yourself. However relaxation is about letting go of tension and focusing on the accompanying feelings in the various muscle groups. Tenseness gives way to sensations like floating, calmness and sometimes tingling which are all signs of relaxation. Mastering this process of relaxation enables the athlete to lower arousal levels and counteract the natural tendency to tense or tighten up when faced with a confrontation.

> 'If you want to win, just relax. There's time for everything.'
>
> *Michael Stich*

A quick and easy way of controlling arousal through relaxation is *ten-point relaxation*. This is illustrated in Figure 11.1 and requires the following circumstances for practice:

- Somewhere *quiet*: though not necessarily needing a soundproof room, distractions should as far as possible be eliminated.
- Get *comfortable*:
  - lying or sitting,
  - head and arms supported,
  - arms and legs uncrossed,
  - loosen tight clothing,
  - remove shoes or trainers,
  - breathe regularly.
- Adopt a *passive attitude*:
  - don't force it, just let it happen,
  - don't think about how well you're doing,
  - if and when your mind wanders, bring your attention back to the exercises.
- Focus on *feeling*:
  - relaxed,
  - warm,
  - calm,
  - heavy.

Ten-point relaxation:

- focus on each muscle group in sequence beginning with '1. Fingers and lower arm' and work through to '10. Entire body';
- spend about one minute on each muscle group;
- eyes closed;
- reflect on how relaxed and heavy the muscles are;
- where tension is noticed, try letting it go by feeling how heavy the muscles can become;
- each time you breathe out, say 'relax' slowly to yourself;
- at the end, open your eyes, feel wide awake and say to yourself 'I'm refreshed, alert and relaxed'.

Athletes need to be able to relax almost instantaneously and sometimes in the heat of competition. The following points help the athlete to gain the ability to relax at will:

- Practise regularly, once a day to begin with.
- Avoid practising immediately after a meal.
- Don't expect too much, too soon.

'I'm working very hard on this relaxation business.'

Graeme Wood

- Try relaxing only one or two of the points – often the neck and shoulders are vulnerable to tension and therefore focus your relaxation on these.
- Relax with your eyes open.
- Say 'relax' to yourself and observe the effect – this often brings on the relaxation response because of the association developed between the word 'relax' and the physical action of letting go.
- Whether sitting, standing, walking or running try to relax different parts of the body.
- Relax non-working muscles during action.

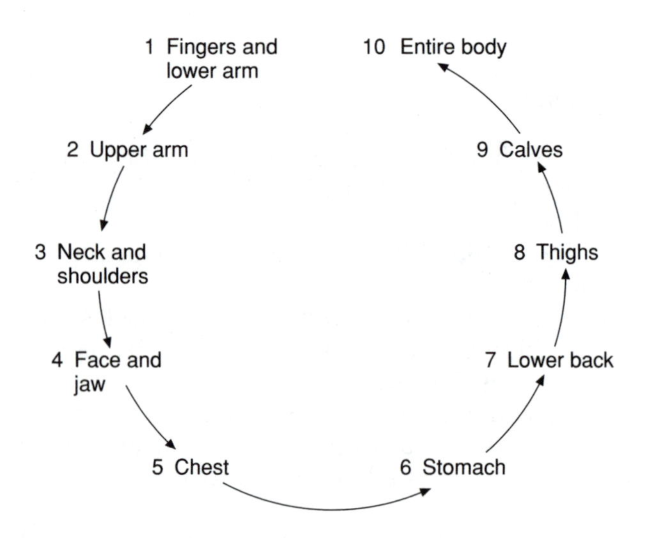

Figure 11.1 Ten-point relaxation

'It's necessary to relax your muscles when you can. Relaxing your brain is fatal.'

Stirling Moss

Relaxation has many uses within sport. It facilitates the control of arousal but it can help the athlete in other ways.

- *Aids sleep* – relaxation enables the muscles to unwind and the focus on heaviness directs the mind away from potentially distracting thoughts and images.
- *Conserves energy* – because relaxation brings about a slowing down of the heart rate, breathing pattern and muscular activity it is ideally employed when energy needs preserving, such as pre-competition and pre-warm-up.
- *Re-vitalizes* – inasmuch as relaxation reduces and erases muscular tension, with athletes reporting the prevention of muscular stiffness, it is usefully employed between events or following hard training sessions or competitions.
- Increases receptiveness – relaxation has an effect on thinking processes, enabling the athlete to approach situations with a clear and open mind. This increases the chance of absorbing information and instructions. A relaxed athlete is more likely therefore to listen to pre-competition team talks and carry through instructions on the field of play. A relaxed athlete is also more likely to benefit from training where it involves the learning of new techniques. Visualization, discussed in the next chapter, is also more inclined to be successful when preceded by relaxation.

'If you control your fear, it makes you more alert, like a deer coming across the lawn.'

Cus D'Amato

12 Visualization

'If ever there was a silent process, it is the creative one.'
Jerome Bruner

Imagine improving a technique without moving a muscle. Sounds improbable, but numerous studies have indeed demonstrated that imagining – picturing yourself in your mind's eye – executing a perfect performance or technique can enhance that skill. Feltz and Landers (1983) even suggest it can, at times, be almost as effective as physically practising the skill. That's the power of visualization.

Visualization appears to be most effective where the following are observed:

- A skill, technique or desired performance is selected.
- Visualization is preceded by *relaxation*. As discussed in Chapter 11, relaxation increases the individual's capacity to absorb information and entertain innovative and fresh ideas. The athlete needs therefore to feel comfortable, close his eyes, regulate his breathing and do a quick 'body scan' for any tension which he then needs to let go.
- Picture the *setting* where the skill in all probability will be performed.
- Exercise all the *senses*. Experience the sounds and smells of the surroundings, the colour, ambience and distinctiveness of the setting as vividly as possible. The most powerful mental images are bright, large, in colour, close up and clear. These features, with practice, can be 'tuned in' so the image is vibrant and lifelike.
- Bring the technique to be worked on into clear *focus*.
- Capture the experience as if you are observing it *through your own eyes*. This is often referred to as an *internal* perspective, which means seeing yourself performing the skill as if physically undertaking it at that time. The alternative is an *external* perspective which is akin to

observing yourself as if you are watching a film. Although top athletes had been thought to typically employ an internal perspective, recent work by Craig Hall and colleagues (Hall, Rodgers and Barr, 1990) suggests they often switch back and forth between internal and external perspectives when imagining themselves performing.

- Attempt to *feel* the movement as it is visualized. This is known as kinesthetic imagery. One advantage of using an internal perspective is that it can facilitate kinesthetic imagery in contrast to an external perspective, which because it relies on seeing the performance from 'outside', cannot include a focus on how the movement feels. Athletes who employ kinesthetic imagery successfully (i.e. they learn to feel the movement during practice) tend to produce successful performances (Mumford and Hall, 1985).
- Try to *perfect* the movement or technique. Craig Hall and his colleagues (Hall *et al.*, 1990) found that kinesthetic imagery may be particularly important for 'closed skills' – those which demand that the athlete undertakes exactly the same movement each time it is performed with perfection being the objective.
- Imagine the skill in the *correct time frame*. No speeded up action or slow motion. Athletes who excel at this leave little margin for error. A 400m runner, for example, can visualize the run to within a second of his personal best.
- Practise visualizing the skill until it feels correct, and try to finish with a perfect performance.

Visualization requires commitment. Regularly practised, as with any other skill, it can begin to make a difference. It makes a difference when practised:

- Alongside and integrated with physical conditioning and technique refinement. Hall and colleagues (Hall *et al.*, 1990) discovered that athletes, even at an elite level, failed to practise regularly and placed less emphasis on planning a session of visualization than they did for other types of training. The coach's role in emphasizing the importance of regular practise, perhaps through designated sessions, then becomes important.

- During periods of inactivity. Athletes may choose to use visualization during times they are prevented from physically participating. Examples include just prior to sleep, when travelling to venues and when injured and out of action.

The array of situations where visualization might prove fruitful include: perfecting a technique, practising the performance, preparing for all eventualities, pre-empting the performance, overcoming difficulties and problems.

Perfecting a technique

In their review of visualization Feltz and Landers (1983) found comprehensive evidence for its effectiveness in facilitating motor skills. However prior physical practice with the skill seems imperative if the visualization is to be effective (Harris and Robinson, 1986). As John Ravey and Deirdre Scully (1989) suggest, if the athlete attempts to visualize a 'new' skill before physically practising the skill, the lack of a prototypic standard against which to evaluate what imagery is appropriate to the task, means superfluous and interfering actions are just as likely to be practised as relevant onces.

The process should therefore incorporate:

- A skill or technique the athlete may be struggling with when practised physically, or one which through visualization can be 'grooved to perfection'.
- Visualization of the skill, identifying the difficulty.
- Practise in imagery a perfect execution of the skill.
- Where this continues to prove formidable, imagine another athlete who excels at the technique and bring into focus their execution of the movement in detail. Then try and imagine being in that athlete's shoes and gradually feel what the movement is like. Practise the perfect accomplishment of the skill with ease.

- Following successful visualization, practise the skill physically.
- Re-play in imagination those skills well accomplished in practice as this will reinforce the movement with a 'visual memory' of the performance.

Practise the performance

Sometimes referred to as 'mental rehearsal' this type of visualization involves running through the desired performance in imagination prior to competition. Of all the types of visualization this is the one most utilized by athletes.

> 'If you want to be a champion, you will have to win every race in your mind one hundred times before you win it in real life, that last time.'
>
> *Marti Liquori*

The process involves:

- gathering as much information as possible about the forthcoming event such as the venue, the course, possible playing conditions, the opposition, your tactical approach and so on;
- in the days prior to performing, run through in your mind's eye the way you intend to perform on the day from start to finish;
- if any aspect feels incorrect, re-run it until you are satisfied it is as good as you can make it;
- as the competition comes closer, begin to include in the visualization those events that precede the competition such as the warm-up, changing room, announcements and so forth.

> 'I did my dives in my head all the time. I started with a front dive, the first one I had to do in the Olympics, and I did everything as if I was actually there. I saw myself on the board preparing for the dive and then performing the dive; if the dive went wrong, I went back and started over again.'
>
> *Sylvie Bernier* (Olympic champion)

> 'The night before a match I would lie in bed and plot what I was going to do on the field the next day. I used to imagine myself pushing the ball between the legs of the defender who I knew would be marking me, and the next day I would go out and do it.'
>
> *George Best*

> 'I'd imagine walking on to the court, tossing for serve, photographers out there ... the night before I'd just run through in my mind and make a checklist of everything I knew about the guy, any titbit of information and then I'd go to sleep.'
>
> *John Newcombe*

Prepare for all eventualities

In addition to mentally rehearsing the desired performance, it can prove useful to prepare, through visualization, for unpredictable events and conditions. This requires imagination in considering possible eventualities and what the best solutions might be. The following quotes will provide a flavour of this type of preparation.

> 'Nothing will be left to chance. You want to know the course so well that you know it by heart. In the end you want to go to sleep at night thinking about it.'
>
> *Nick Faldo*

> 'I would walk up to the back of the stands and look down on the court and I'd imagine my arms enveloping the net posts and the court, and I'd close my eyes and have a mental picture of the court and myself being one – familiarity, so that when I came to play there I felt right at home.'
>
> *John Newcombe*

Pre-empt the performance

This form of visualization is undertaken during breaks in competition where the desired action is visualized just prior to the performance. It lends itself very naturally to the following sports and situations:

- Where there are a succession of repeated routines or perfected plays e.g. weight-lifting; gymnastics; diving;

high jump; long/triple jump; shot; hammer; javelin; discus; archery; shooting.

- Where there is a break prior to performing an action e.g. serving in badminton, squash, tennis; bowling in cricket; pitching; shots in snooker and golf; free throw in basketball; darts; bowls; penalties in football, hockey and rugby.
- Where the start is all important e.g. bobsleigh; sprints; skiing.

The process is as follows:

- Take a breather, using the centering technique and relax the shoulders and neck.
- Picture the action as you want it to happen, visualizing the performance from start to finish.
- Where possible enhance the target or objective. This counteracts the tendency, when anxious, to perceive objects as smaller than they are in actuality. For example, imagine an increase in the size of the basket, pocket or hole.
- Visualize the performance as successful.
- Take a breather and attempt the action.

Pre-empting performance in this way appears to have a number of positive effects. It encourages the athlete to stay focused as the desired performance is the object of the visualization; it strengthens self belief because the athlete anticipates a successful accomplishment of the performance; and finally it tends to help the athlete control arousal level because the focus is internal.

> 'I always visualize my putting stroke as an attempt to drive an imaginary tack into the back of a ball.'
>
> *Walter Travis*

Overcome difficulties and problems

In addition to assisting athletes to improve their performance, visualization may also find favour where troublesome issues need confronting:

- *Overcoming error tendencies.* Graham Jones (1993) described how visualization helped an athlete effectively deal with anger following errors made by both herself or the official. The athlete was encouraged to reconstruct under imagery the tendency to become angry and then to re-structure a more desired or preferred reaction which was in turn visualized until the athlete felt able to respond in this way.
- *Overcoming anticipated difficulties.* Situations can feel threatening when the athlete is unsure about how they will handle a situation such as giving an interview to the press, approaching the coach with a personal problem or feeling their way into the culture of a new team. Visualizing a scenario where the athlete confronts the difficulty with a degree of success can dramatically increase the individual's ability to deal with the event.
- *Overcoming self-defeating expectations.* Sometimes athletes will set a standard, expectation or goal far below their potential. Harry Stanton (1992) described what he called the 'swish technique' which assists athletes to change self-fulfilling prophecies. The example Stanton gives is of a sprinter who in training often ran faster times than the competitors she faced but rarely beat them in competition. The 'swish technique' as applied to this sprinter goes as follows:
  - Identify the context (the preponderance of second placings).
  - Develop a cue picture – the image of now things are at the moment seen from an internal perspective (the back of another girl breasting the tape in front of her).
  - Develop an outcome picture – the desired image (running smoothly, striding away from her opponents, breasting the tape ahead of the other runners).
  - Now imagine the cue picture big and bright filling the mind (vivid details of the girl in front such as damp tendrils of hair and the play of muscles.)
  - In a lower corner of this image mentally place a small dark image of the desired outcome.
  - This small desired image is mentally 'zoomed' so that it quickly grows bright and enlarges to cover completely the first picture which vanishes. This

process must be fast, taking a couple of seconds at most.

- The eyes are opened.
- The swish is repeated five times.
- Effectiveness is tested by trying to imagine the original cue picture – the athlete should find this difficult to do without it quickly zooming into the desired action.

13 Cope with pressure

'Pressure does crazy things to athletes. Some love it, thrive on it, others choke on it. Most learn to live with it.'

Herman L. Masin

This quote elucidates a core principle concerning pressure. Although it is often understood that the environment or circumstances create pressure, these 'external' events can only create the context, not the pressure. The experience of pressure or stress comes from the athlete's *perception* of the event, not the event itself. A similar event may evoke feelings of stress or excitement depending upon how the athlete construes the environment.

Given such a framework, this chapter covers:

- events which have the potential for generating a feeling of stress or pressure,
- means by which the athlete might cope with situations that are construed as stressful.

Potentially stressful events

Some events clearly have features which athletes are, on the whole, more likely to construe negatively or stressfully. Those events which arise unpredictably such as changes in playing conditions or injury, were discussed in Chapter 6. This chapter reviews more predictable events, particularly those that accompany more 'important' competition. Important here means not only those events faced by athletes at an elite level where competition is undertaken predominantly in the limelight, but also those competitions, faced by athletes of all abilities, which carry a higher status (e.g. a final; a local derby; a trial) or assume personal significance for an individual (e.g. a debut).

A survey of potentially stressful events would include:

- travel to the competition – long distances, delays, waiting for connections;
- extra bureaucracy – correspondence, accreditation, security, queues;
- boredom – perhaps with a tendency to do extra training, over-eating or nibbling; becoming homesick;
- unfamiliar accommodation – uncomfortable beds, over-crowding, sharing conveniences;
- spectators – autograph seekers, hangers-on, hostile crowds;
- organizational hiccups – delays, changes, lack of available information;
- the media – intrusions, high expectations, insatiable demands.

Coping with pressure

P *prepare*
R *relax*
E *externalize*
S *stay positive*
S *single minded*
U *unite*
R *re-evaluate*
E *extend yourself*

Prepare

'The mind is something to think with, not just for worrying.'
Anonymous

Athletes need to prepare, or 'acclimatize psychologically' for what they will be faced with. Preparation can take many forms:

- Simulate the event, or features of the event, (e.g. role playing an interview with the press) as far as it is possible prior to the competition. This increases a sense of familiarization and belief in ability to cope.

- Visualize situations which are potentially stressful. This further validates the athlete's ability to deal with the situation effectively.
- Control the controllables. This may mean taking very practical precautions such as games to alleviate boredom, personal photos to personalize the room, a Walkman to use when waiting or queuing, a pillow to help sleep, favourite cereals or chocolate bars.
- Find out from experienced athletes how they manage the pressure effectively.
- Develop a strategy, which guides how the athlete is expected to behave in a given situation.

Terry Orlick (1986) has discussed the development of a strategy related in particular to facing the media. He suggests one of the most important actions a team can take in preparing for competition is to establish a 'media protocol' which every member of the team is involved in developing and as a result each member understands how to act in the situation. Orlick suggests the following should be considered in developing the plan or protocol:

- A 'press kit', giving essential details of the athlete(s), released to the press prior to any interview so reporters are informed.
- Control the schedule and tell the press in advance what this schedule will be. The team may wish to hold a pre-competition interview/session a few days before competition and not again until after the event. This protects the athlete(s) from being overwhelmed or constantly distracted by media requests.
- A clear demarcation of when the athlete will not be available to the media. Thus an athlete might choose not to give interviews prior to training, at the competition site or on the day of competition.
- An outline of when coaches and support staff will be available to the press, which might vary from the players in order to 'protect' the team from unwelcome intrusions or exposure.
- How the athlete should react when approached 'off limits'. Orlick provides the following example as a

preplanned response: 'I'm sorry but there is a team policy, and as such I can't talk now but I will be available after the event in the finish area'.

- How the athlete can best put himself across. The following are some pointers:
  - speak slowly (when nervous we tend to speed up),
  - smile,
  - be yourself; open, honest and personable,
  - use gestures, especially hands which express your feeling and counteracts stiffness,
  - answer the question,
  - ensure you get across the main points,
  - be aware of outcome questions (e.g. 'are you going to win today?') because the danger is that the athlete starts to think in this way rather than focusing on performance goals.

> 'Facing the press is more difficult than bathing a leper.'
>
> *Mother Teresa*

Relax

Relaxation, in its many forms, employed during the duration of a competition or prior to a stressful event will enable the athlete to remain in control and ease or prevent muscular tension developing. Types of relaxation athletes have found useful, listed in approximate order of how quickly they can be implemented are:

- cue words e.g. 'calm', 'relax',
- centering,
- localized relaxation (especially neck and shoulders),
- ten-point relaxation,
- listening to music,
- massage.

Externalize

> 'Half the battle with stress is thinking you're under stress.'
>
> *Ian Botham*

Externalization is the belief (although not necessarily the expression) that the problem lies not within yourself but with someone else. This is a form of defence or self protection but it can prove useful when other people are making excessive demands on your time and energy. In practice the athlete might be helped to see that:

- Criticism is the *opinion* of another, not a fact, and that people who criticise commit 'professional fouls' because they go for the man, not the ball (i.e. they tend to attack the person not the performance).
- Unreasonable demands from others (e.g. for interviews) implies that the problem lies with them, not you (e.g. they have a story to compile). They are like used car salesmen who have a problem and try to offload that onto someone else.

Stay positive

'People who feel good perform better.'

Frank Dick

The important thing, no matter how difficult the situation, is to maintain the belief in yourself. Confidence transmits itself to others including team mates and competitors. Team mates will profit; competitors will perhaps be intimidated. Self belief strategies were discussed in Chapter 9. Emphasis on performance accomplishments seems the key to maintaining confidence. Some examples of what the athlete may focus on when 'threatened' by potentially stressful events are:

- 'I've done it before; this is no different.'
- 'I'd been picked; therefore I can do the job.'
- 'I've prepared for this; now go and do it.'
- 'Get my performance right and the result will take care of itself.'
- 'This is my chance; seize it.'

Single minded

'The secret is not to let outside factors register.'

Geoff Boycott

Important competitions increase the spectrum of potential distractions. There are build-up distractors (e.g. local and national coverage; interviews; money-raising functions), on-site distractors (e.g. entertainment; socializing; tourist attractions; sunbathing; using new facilities), and finally the outcome is given greater prominence (e.g. the prestige of being champion; eminence and reputation riding on the result).

Maintaining an appropriate focus has to be paramount if the athlete is to 'ride' the pressure and perform well. Temptations have to be avoided until after the event. The focus should be on:

- achieving quality in whatever the athlete does (training, resting, preparing equipment, giving an interview);
- concentrating on what needs to be done in order to perform well (e.g. diet, relaxation, planning);
- performance issues, not the outcome or ramifications of possible success.

Unite

> 'The whole is greater than the sum of its parts.'
>
> *Anonymous*

This concept, concerning how the individual relates to the team, has three elements: the unit, a unity and being united.

The *unit*: wherever possible there seem to be advantages in the team operating as a unit. The old adage of 'strength in numbers' expresses the sentiment. Having each member of the team dressed similarly in tracksuit, training kit, leisure wear or formal wear expresses the solidarity of the team in addition to providing a sense of identity for individual members of the team. A team attending functions or training as a unit also establishes purpose, pride and commitment for the individuals involved. The messages conveyed (and therefore sensed by the team members in addition to onlookers including other competitors) by a group of athletes behaving as a unit include power, domination, authority and potency.

A *unity*: teams maintain or develop a distinctive culture which each individual must feel a part of, for the team to have harmony and an agreement to pursue a single purpose. There is a careful balance to achieve within a team for the unity to evolve. There needs to be a team goal – a mission statement about what the team is aiming to achieve – developed and agreed by all individuals within the team. Each individual then needs to be clear about tasks that are required of him in pursuing the team goal and further, given the responsibility to carry them through. Such team harmony and the support individuals receive through their combined efforts, in many ways buffer the individual athlete from potentially stressful times. This does not apply exclusively to sports played as a team, but to all sports, given that even those undertaken individually will usually perform alongside colleagues and under a team 'umbrella'.
Being united: Within a team individuals play roles. Informally a leader will emerge, alongside a joker, a man of ideas and someone who does things by the book. When this gels, team spirit transpires. However more formal roles may also be demanded if the team is to function successfully. Effective teams decide who will deal with what. Essential tasks are identified from checking kit and equipment to checking kick-off times, from team selection to counselling dropped or injured athletes, from making a dossier of future opponents to dealing with requests from the media. Some tasks may cut across professional boundaries but what should remain paramount in deciding who does what, is how the team and the individual members of that team will benefit.

Re-evaluate

> 'If you play as if it means nothing when it means everything, you've got it.'
>
> *Steve Davis*

This is an attempt to negate the appraisal of the event as necessarily important. When events assume enormous proportions in the thinking of athletes, they tend to underperform, become anxious and sometime 'crumble'. An option to consider, no matter how important the event, is this: 'it's the same me, competing in the same event, an event I've done many times before and quite successfully, so I know I can do well'. This focuses again on the performance, and the individual's self efficacy rather than the event.

Extend yourself

> 'The only limitations are mental. The guy who thinks positively will win.'
>
> *Daley Thompson*

Committing yourself to perform at your best was covered in Chapter 4. Pressures in some ways can be seen as challenges – they provide the opportunity to test yourself, sometimes to the limit. An interesting task is to consider the advantages of coping with the demands imposed by potentially stressful situations. Giving press interviews for example, provide the opportunity of gaining recognition for the sport you are involved in as well as providing an opportunity to educate others on some of the finer points of your event. If athletes can construe pressure in the way Billie Jean King did, then it no longer is pressure. She once remarked 'I like pressure, the challenge – it's exciting.'

14 Strategy

'The only way to predict the future is to have power to shape the future.'

Eric Hoffer

Ultimately the measure of how well an athlete will perform is determined by the degree to which he is able to make the potentially unpredictable, predictable. The theme running through the previous chapters has been enhancing the athlete's capacity to generate accomplished and consistent performances. Performances which do the athlete justice irrespective of the conditions or the circumstances the athlete finds himself in. The final piece of the 'jigsaw' is placing this within the context of competition given the uniqueness of each particular sporting event. This requires strategy, a blueprint of desired action which takes account of exceptional factors and anticipated possibilities. A strategy should therefore facilitate and guide a performance to meet the demands of each specific performance.

Strategies are plans to guide action. They can typically be divided into:

- pre-competition plans,
- competition plans or tactics, and
- post-competition plans, or analysis.

Pre-competition plans

'I used to work backwards from the time I wanted to be able to sit down with a nice cup of tea and give myself a short break before the match began ... as a matter of habit I arrived on the ground an hour and a half before the start of play, leaving myself ten minutes to get changed, fifty minutes for exercise and a net, and thirty minutes to cool down and think through what the day might have in store.'

Geoff Boycott

In many respects Geoff Boycott says it all. His schedule was presumably evolved through experience to become a habit, almost a ritual in itself, which facilitated Boycott achieving a perfect state of readiness prior to competition. This type of planning is formalized in Figure 14.1 which can be employed to help athletes begin thinking about how they might design or plan the best way of utilizing the final hours before competition. The final hours can prove vital. Having a predetermined plan provides a familiar routine, a performance focus and a sense of control. The plan is concerned with building a sequence of actions which enhance the athlete's readiness. Using Figure 14.1 to record the athlete's responses, the following questions will increasingly help build up the plan:

- What are the deadlines; the times which have to be met that day:
  - start or kick-off time;
  - assemble time for team;
  - practise time;
  - warm-up time;
- What is specific to this competition which has to be built in to the plan:
  - travel arrangements
- What must the athlete ensure happens:
  - morning alarm
  - pack kit and equipment
- What does the athlete wish to do that will enable him to feel best prepared; this might include things which have previously been found to work:
  - what to eat and when to eat
  - relaxation
  - mental rehearsal
  - clarification of tactics with coach

The complete time schedule should preferably be filled in so the athlete is not left with gaps and consequently time on his hands. A further important aspect of developing a pre-competition plan, as suggested by Brent Rushall (1979) is to prepare an alternative strategy or plan in the event of unplanned delays or interruptions to the schedule. Figure 14.1 provides a column for 'alternative plans' which gives the athlete a feeling of control even when original plans are disrupted.

A particular form of pre-competition behaviour which remains constant and generates a sense of control for the athlete is the ritual.

> 'I put my left shinpad on first, put my right boot and my right glove on first ... I always go through that routine.'
>
> *Chris Woods* (goalkeeper)

Event:...

Time	Plan	Alternative

Start →

Figure 14.1 Schedule for developing pre-competition strategies

Rituals are the expression of superstitions. A superstition is a belief that a certain way of acting will produce a desired result. Thus kit bags are packed in particular ways, getting changed is undertaken in a specific sequence, lucky attire is worn, driving a distinct route to the ground becomes the norm, eating a specific meal before playing, are all embarked on because sometime in the past such an action became associated with a successful performance or outcome. A ritual is the routine or behaviour the athlete goes through to satisfy the superstition.

When a ritual is followed by a good performance, the superstition is validated thus increasing the likelihood that the athlete will act that way in the future. Even a series of poor performances will often not invalidate the superstition because the belief is held so strongly. Sometimes the ritual will even increase following a poor performance because the athlete may attribute the poor performance to inefficient undertaking of the ritual, therefore vowing to ensure the ritual is better executed during the next performance.

Rituals can be construed as providing structure, much like a pre-competition plan, in the face of uncertainty. As such they may be perceived as ways of establishing control during preparation and can further act as time markers as the competition approaches.

> 'I always try to go out after the number 9 shirt. I don't know why, but I've been doing it for years.'
>
> *Steve McMahon*

Tactics

> 'A captain must always make his decisions before he knows what will happen. The critic usually bases his statement on what has happened and thus takes no risk.'
>
> *Sir Don Bradman*

The quote by Don Bradman aptly touches on the fundamental issues in relation to tactical endeavours. There is the concept of anticipation – a prediction of how the event might unfold; decision making and planning to structure performance to achieve a particular purpose; and finally the notion of risk taking which may influence the plans that are hatched.

The process of tactical planning may involve some or all of the following aspects:

Exploration of the situation

1) *Analysis of the athlete or team strengths.* This can involve gathering the athlete and team's ideas of what they consider to be their strengths through discussion or performance profiling (Chapter 2), in addition to accumulating ideas from coaches and support staff. A tactical approach might be based exclusively on applying such perceived strengths. Examples might be relying on a fast start, a tight defence, a powerful first serve, irregular changes of tempo and so forth.
2) *Analyse the opponent's strengths and vulnerabilities.* Many examples exist of 'dossiers' being collated on future competitors. The key is to look for replications in the way they behave or perform within and between different events. This supplies information on relatively stable ways the opponents behave and thus it would be predicted, especially when under pressure, that they would consistently behave in this fashion. Ways of exposing and taking advantages of vulnerabilities then have to be considered, alongside ways to counteract their strengths. Alan Border, the Australian cricket captain, studied in detail how opposing batsmen tended to make their runs and what their preferred shots were, subsequently and very effectively setting specified fields to thwart their capacity to make runs.

'He does a lot of things wrong, but right now there's nobody around who can take advantage of these things.'

Angela Dundee on Mike Tyson

3) *Analyse the conditions.* Whilst taking into account the particular features of a competition (e.g. the weather, the draw, the playing surface) which have to be assessed in relation to how they can best be utilized to the athlete's advantage (as discussed in Chapter 6) there

may be some facets of the sport which can be actively manipulated to advantage. This may require detailed analysis of particular plays with video playback, note-book or research method. Sometimes it seems almost to be folklore within the sport. For example the vulnerability of a football team having just scored, to conceding a goal in the next few minutes, because of a lapse of concentration, is well known. Reference to literature on the sport can also be illuminating. Charles Hughes, for example, did a detailed analysis of football and discovered the biggest single factor in scoring goals is set plays; the biggest factor in winning set plays is free kicks; and the biggest factor in getting free kicks is dribbling with the ball and taking on defenders. Such information might prove invaluable in assessing how the athlete or team might best profit from the situation.

4) *Examine the current parameters of play.* All sports have rules which are relatively fluid i.e. they are constantly being adapted and changed. With any change comes opportunity. A new rule offers a challenge, a means of exploring fresh ways of taking an advantage. Perhaps the most famous example of a loophole in sport being taken advantage of was bodyline bowling which emerged in cricket as a tactic to 'remove' Don Bradman. By packing the leg side with fielders and bowling fast and short down the leg side it was hoped that any tendency to play at the ball would result in a catch for the fielders. This tactic caused an international row and subsequent rule changes to prevent it happening again. It also illustrates the moral dilemma faced by a coach wishing to exercise an advantage which might test the rules of the sport. The power of innovation must be allowed to prosper but care has to be taken not to cross the moral boundary – the unwritten rules that have evolved for the necessary smooth running of the sport.

Decision making

Given an assessment of the athlete or team strengths, the opponent's strengths and vulnerabilities, the advantages to be gained in the current situation and any innovations inspired by the games' laws, the next steps are to decide on:

1) *The risk.* The chances of success have, of course, to outweigh the possibility of failure. Further risks involve when to employ the tactic as 'showing your cards' too early, too late or if well in front or too far behind, will reduce the impact.
2) *How to employ the tactic.* For maximum effect the following might be considered:
   - Taking *control* wherever possible through changing the predominant set or rhythm so that you 'dictate' the terms. e.g. changing tempo, changing the pace, calling a time out, making a substitution. This might cause opponents to alter or adjust their preferred game plan.
   - being *unpredictable* so that opponents feel unable to anticipate your moves, which may cause opponents to shift focus so they are no longer attending to their own performance.

'You just never know what he's up to and it psyches you out.'

Bob Kreiss on Ille Nastase

   - *Camouflage* intentions by disguising your plans or even giving up what appears to be an advantage for a longer-term success.

'It's all so much a mental thing. You've got to make the other person curl up more.'

Elvis Gordon

Analysis

'It's easy to do anything in victory. It's in defeat that a man reveals himself.'

Floyd Patterson

This quote does not imply that successful performances should not be analysed. Clearly all performances offer the opportunity to discover new facets of the athlete. What poor performances tend to do however, is create detrimental emotional experiences which cloud an objective assessment. The initial reaction to a poor performance should therefore be consolation and an effort to put it in context. Self worth is not determined by the outcome of a performance, and the athlete should therefore never feel he is less of a person because of a poor performance. Perhaps some of the best illustrations of putting 'defeat' in context are the following compelling quotes:

> 'What's baseball when compared to death? What's baseball compared to starvation? It's a game.'
>
> *Jose Canesco*

> 'I'm not immortal. I didn't lose a war. Nobody died. I only lost a tennis match.'
>
> *Boris Becker*

> 'No matter what happens, I can always dig ditches for a living.'
>
> *Arnold Palmer*

> 'Winning or not winning is not so important. It is only a transient moment in life.'
>
> *Ayrton Senna*

Sandy Gordon (1990) uses what he terms 'the four Rs' in post-game analysis – review, retain, rest and return. With some adaptation this format is acknowledged as a fruitful means of conducting a de-brief which seeks to use the experience of the latest performance to help in preparing for the next performance.

Review

> 'The path of a successful sportsman is never a smooth one.'
>
> *Jack Fingleton*

A review of the last performance might take place a day or two following the competition in order that it can be analysed reasonably objectively and free of emotional reactions associated with it. The review stage is essentially data gathering, collected in the following ways:

1) By seeking responses to the following questions:
   - What went well?
   - What was accomplished or achieved?
   - How did the performance compare with a previous best?
   - Did the performance match the game plan?
   - What surprised you about the performance?
   - What were you disappointed with?

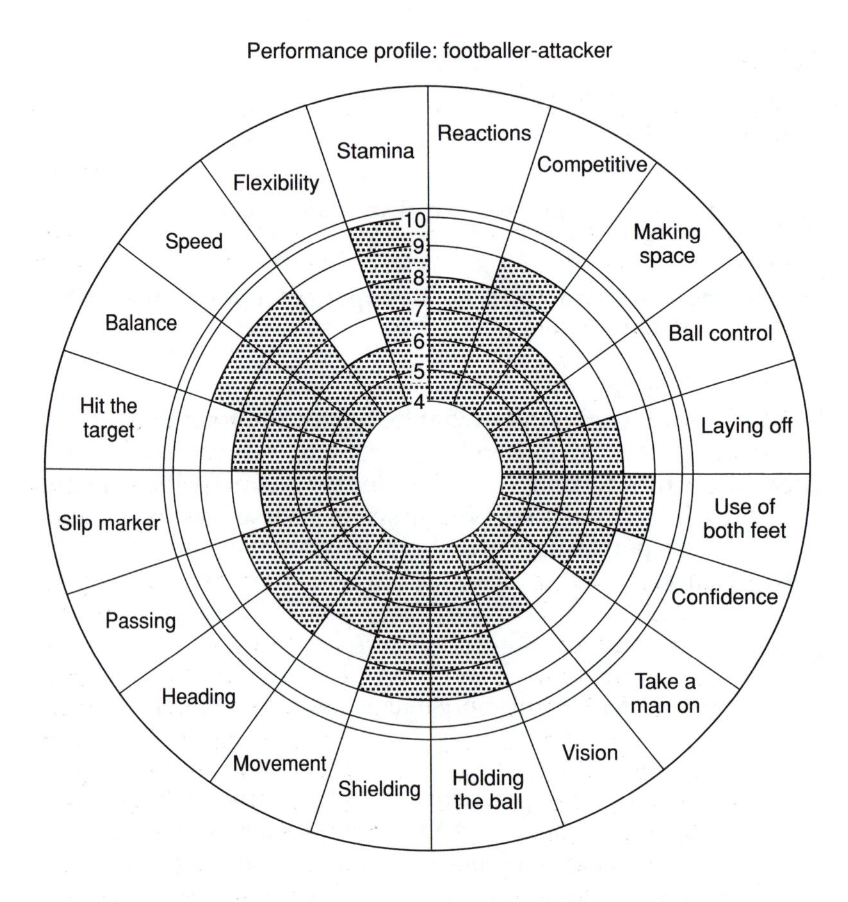

Figure 14.2 Post-match assessment

2) By undertaking a performance profile as a post-match assessment. Figure 14.2 provides an example of such an assessment with a football player. The qualities considered important for the footballer to perform well are placed on the perimeter and the player rates his latest performance on each quality. This provides a visual display of how the athlete experienced his performance. It highlights those areas where the player considered he did well (shielding, stamina, use of both feet and so forth) and those areas which he felt were not satisfactory (flexibility, taking a man on).

Reflect

> 'An athlete who fails is one who does not maximize the use of their potential, not necessarily one who loses a race.'
>
> *Cliff Temple*

This step is concerned with discussion, elaboration and reflection of the information with a view to analysing the changes that need to be made prior to the next performance. Some ways this might be facilitated are:

1) Establishing what needs to be done differently.
2) Deciding what has to be put in place for the athlete to perform at his best.
3) Confirm ways the athlete did himself justice; which goals were achieved and how can these be consolidated.
4) Discover, if possible, unstable reasons for a poor performance, but reasons which acknowledge the athlete's responsibility. This usually means attributing poor performances to *unstable* but *controllable* factors (such as lack of effort, a dip in form) which are possible to change. Attributing poor performance to stable or uncontrollable factors (such as lack of ability, poor refereeing decisions, difficult conditions) are more difficult to change and should therefore be avoided.

   An example of an attribute shift occurred in the film *Chariots of Fire* when Harold Abrahams, after losing to Eric Liddle, said 'I did my best. I was beaten by a better man. I can't run any faster.' (a stable and defeating attribute). To this his girlfriend added 'today' (an unstable attribute allowing for the possibility of change). Following this encounter Abrahams did concentrate on improving his efforts and ultimately went on to win Olympic gold.

5) With the performance profile (Figure 14.2), the coach may also rate the athlete independently on the same qualities, feeding this back to the athlete so he is able to see how the coach feels about the performance. Where a large discrepancy arises between the athlete and coach's ratings on any quality, the issues and information on which each rating was based should be discussed so that an understanding is reached and subsequently acted on.

Rest

The recovery phase. Relaxation, massage or sauna are effective means of assisting the body to recover from exercise. This phase may however also be profitably used to consolidate any proposed changes through practising visualization.

Re-editing is a visualization technique best suited to this phase of the de-brief. It consists of:

- visualizing the performance, or element of performance that was performed inadequately,
- re-editing the visualization so the performance is completed as it ideally should be,
- practising the re-edited visualization regularly.

Return

The successful athlete returns with renewed vigour, enthusiasm, appetite and a re-formulated game plan, modified via the post-match analysis and subsequently tested and perfected through both physical and psychological training.

> 'Winners are those that do their best. They don't necessarily win gold medals.'
>
> *Dick Jochurns*

References

BANDURA, A. (1977) 'Self efficacy: towards a unifying theory of behavioural change.' *Psychological Review*, **84**, 191–215.

BANNISTER, D. and FRANSELLA, F. (1986) *Inquiring Man: The Psychology of Personal Constructs*. Croom Helm, London.

BIDDLE, S. J. H. (1986) 'Personal beliefs and mental preparation in strength and muscular endurance tasks: a review'. *Physical Education Review*, **8**, 90–103.

BULL, S. J., FLEMING, S. and DOUST, J. (1992) *Play better cricket: Using sport science to improve your game*. Sport Dynamics, Eastbourne.

BURTON, D. (1989) 'Winning isn't everything: Examining the impact of peformance goals on collegiate swimmers' cognitions and performance.' *The Sport Psychologist*, **3**, 105–132.

BUTLER, R. J. (1989) 'Psychological preparation of Olympic boxers'. In J. Kremer and W. Crawford (eds) *The Psychology of Sport: Theory and practice*. BPS, Leicester.

BUTLER, R. J. (in press) 'Applying psychological principles to sports injuries.' In S. French (ed.) Physiotherapy: A Psychological Approach. Oxford, Butterworth-Heinemann.

BUTLER, R. J. and HARDY, L. (1992) 'The performance profile: Theory and application'. *The Sport Psychologist*, **6**, 253–264.

BUTLER, R. J., SMITH, M. and IRWIN, L. (1993) The performance profile in practice. *J. Applied Sport Psychology*, **5**, 48–63.

COX, R. J. (1995) 'Individual intervention: The fall and rise of a professional golfer'. In R. J. Butler (ed) *Sport Psychology in Performance*. Butterworth-Heinemann, Oxford.

FELTZ, D. L. (1982) 'A path analysis of the causal elements in Bandura's theory of self-efficacy and anxiety based model of avoidance behaviour.' *J. of Personality and Social Psychology*, **42**, 764–781.

FELTZ, D. L. and DOYLE, L. A. (1981) 'Improving self-confidence in athletic performance'. *Motor Skills: Theory into Practice*, **5**, 89–96.

FELTZ, D. L. and LANDERS, D. (1983) 'The effects of mental practice on motor skill learning and performance: a meta analysis'. *J. Sport Psychology*, **5**, 25–57.
FELTZ, D. L. and MUGNO, D. A. (1983) 'A replication of the path analysis of the causal elements in Bandura's theory of self efficacy and and the influence of autonomic perception'. *J. Sports Psychology*, **5**, 161–277.
FELTZ, D. L. and WEISS, M. R. (1982) 'Developing self efficacy through sport.' *J. Physical Education, Recreation & Dance*, **53**, 24–26.
GALLWEY, W. T. (1974) *The Inner Game of Tennis*. Bantam, New York.
GARFIELD, C. A. and BENNETT, H. A. (1984) *Peak Performance: Mental Training Techniques of the World's Greatest Athletes*. Tarcher, Los Angeles.
GARLAND, H. (1985) 'A cognitive mediation of task goals and human performance'. *Motivation & Emotion*, **9**, 345–367.
GAURON, E. F. (1984) *Mental Training for Peak Performance*. Lansing, Sport Science Associates, New York.
GORDON, S. (1990) 'A mental skills training programme for the Western Australian state cricket team'. *The Sport Psychologist*, **4**, 386–399.
GOULD, D., HODGE, K., PETERSON, K. and GIANNINI, J. (1989) 'An exploratory examination of strategies used by elite coaches to enhance self efficacy in athletes'. *J. Sport & Exercise Psychology*, **11**, 128–140.
GOULD, D., EKLUND, R. C. and JACKSON, S. A. (1992a) '1988 U.S. Olympic wrestling excellence: 1 mental preparation, precompetitive cognition and affect'. *The Sport Psychologist*, **6**, 358–382.
GOULD, D., EDKLUND, R. C. and JACKSON, S. A. (1992b) '1988 U.S. Olympic wrestling excellence: 2 thoughts and affect occurring during competition'. *The Sport Psychologist*, **6**, 383–402.
GOULD, D. and UDRY, E. (1994) 'Psychological skills for enhancing performance: arousal regulation strategies. *Medicine & Science in Sport and Exercise*, 478–485.
GROVE, J. R. and PRAPAVESSIS, H. (1992) 'Preliminary evidence for the reliability and validity of an abbreviated profile of mood states'. *Int. J. Sport Psychology*, **23**, 93–109.

HALL, C. R., RODGERS, W. M. and BARR, K. A. (1990) 'The use of imagery by athletes in selected sports'. *The Sport Psychologist*, **4**, 1–10.
HARDY, L. (1990) 'A catastrophe model of performance in sport'. In J. G. Jones and L. Hardy (eds) *Stress and Performance in Sport*. Wiley, Chichester.
HARRIS, D. V. and ROBINSON, W. J. (1986) 'The effect of skill level on EMG activity during internal and external imagery. *J. Sport Psychology*, **8**, 105–111.
HEMERY, D. (1991) *Sporting Excellence*. Collins Willow, London.
HIGHLEN, P. S. and BENNETT, B. B. (1979) 'Psychological characteristics of successful and non-successful elite wrestlers: an exploratory study. *J. Sport Psychology*, **1**, 123–137.
JONES, G. (1993) 'The role of performance profiling in cognitive behavioural interventions in sport'. *The Sport Psychologist*, **7**, 160–172.
KERR, G. and FOWLER, B. (1988) 'The relationship between psychological factors and sports injuries'. *Sports Medicine*, **6**, 127–134.
KUBISTANT, T. (1986) *Performing your Best*. Human Kinetics, Champaign, Illinois.
McCOY, M. M. (1977) 'The reconstruction of emotion'. In D. Bannister (ed) *New Perspectives in Personal Construct Theory*. Academic Press, London.
MAHONEY, M. J. (1979) 'Cognitive skills and athletic performance'. In P. C. Kendall and S. D. Hollon (eds) *Cognitive – Behavioural Interventions: Theory, Research and Procedures*. Academic Press, New York.
MAHONEY, M. J. and AVENER, M. (1977) 'Psychology of the elite athlete: an exploratory study'. *Cognitive Therapy & Resarch*, **1**, 135–142.
MORGAN, W. P. (1979) 'Prediction of performance in athletics'. In P. Klavora and J. V. Daniel (eds) *Coach, Athlete and the Sport Psychologist*. Human Kinetics, Champaign, Illinois.
MORGAN, W. P., BROWN, D. R., RAGLIN, J. S., O'CONNOR, P. J., ELLICKSON, K. A. (1987) 'Psychological monitoring of overtraining and staleness'. *Brit J. Sports Medicine*, **21**, 107–114.

MUMFORD, B. and HALL, C. (1985) 'The effects of internal and external imagery on performing figures in figure skating'. *Canadian J. of Applied Sport Science*, **10**, 171–177.
NIDEFFER, R. M. (1976) 'Test of attentional and interpersonal style'. *J. of Personality and Social Psychology*, **34**, 394–404.
O'HAGAN, S. and MAUME, C. (1994) *The Independent Book of Sports Questions and Answers*. Boxtree, London.
ORLICK, T. (1986) *Psyching for Sport*. Leisure Press, Champaign, Illinois.
ORLICK, T. (1990) *In Pursuit of Excellence*. Leisure Press, Champaign, Illinois.
ORLICK, T. and PARTINGTON, J. (1988) 'Mental links to excellence'. *The Sports Psychologist*, **2**, 105–130.
RAVEY, J. and SCULLY, D. (1989) 'The cognitive psychology of sport'. In J. Kremer and W. Crawford (eds) *The Psychology of Sport: Theory and Practice*. BPS, Leicester.
RAVIZZA, K. (1977) 'Peak experience in sport'. *J. Humanistic Psychology*, **17**, 35–40.
RAVIZZA, K. (1987) 'The integration of psychological skills training into practice sessions'. In J. H. Salmela (ed) *Psychological Nuturing and Guidance of Gymnastic Talent*. Sport Psyche Editions, Montreal.
RAVIZZA, K. and OSBORNE, T. (1991) 'Nebraska's 3 R's: One play at a time preperformance routine for collegiate football'. *The Sport Psychologist*, **5**, 256–265.
RUSHALL, B. S. (1979). *Psyching for Sport*. Pelham, London.
SCANLAN, T. K., CARPENTER, P. J., SHMIDT, G. W., SIMONS, J. P. and KEELER, B. (1993) 'An introduction to the sport commitment model'. *J. Sport & Exercise Psychology*, **151**, 1–15.
SCHACHAM, S. (1983) 'A shortened version of the Profile of Mood States'. *J. Personality Assessment*, **47**, 305–306.
SHELTON, T. O. and MAHONEY, M. J. (1978) 'The content and effect of "psyching up" strategies in weightlifters'. *Cognitive Therapy & Research*, **2**, 275–284.
SMITH, A. M., SCOTT, S. G. and WEISE, D. M. (1990) 'The psychological effects of sports injuries'. *Sports Medicine*, **9**, 352–369.
STANTON, H. E. (1992) 'Improving sporting performance through brief therapy'. *Excel*, **8**, 191–195.
SYER, J. (1989) *Team Spirit*. Simon & Schuster, London.

SYER, J. and CONNOLLY, C. (1984). *Sporting Body, Sporting Mind*. Cambridge University Press, Cambridge.
TERRY, P. (1989) *The Winning Mind*. Thorsons, Wellingborough.
WEINBERG, R. (1994) 'Goal setting and performance in sport and exercise settings: a synthesis and critique'. *Medicine and Science in Sports and Exercise*, 469–477.
WEINBERG, R. S., GOULD, D. and JACKSON, A. (1979) 'Expectations and performance: an empirical test of Bandura's self efficacy theory'. *J. Sport Psychology*, **1**, 320–331.
WEISS, M. R. and TROXELL, R. K. (1986) 'Psychology of the injured athlete'. *Athletic Training*, **154**, 104–109.
WIESE, D. M. and WEISS, M. R. (1987) 'Psychological rehabilitation and physical injury: implications for the sports medicine team'. *The Sport Psychologist*, **1**, 318–330.

Index